Advanced Therapies in Pediatric Endocrinology and Diabetology

With an unrestricted educational grant from

Pfizer

Università di Roma Tor Vergata

Bambino Gesù OSPEDALE PEDIATRICO

SCUOLA DI PEDIATRIA

Master di II Livello in Endocrinologia e Diabetologia Pediatrica – Scuola di Pediatria

# Endocrine Development

**Vol. 30**

Series Editor

P.-E. Mullis Bern

Workshop, Rome, October 27–28, 2014

# Advanced Therapies in Pediatric Endocrinology and Diabetology


Volume Editors

Marco Cappa Rome

Stefano Cianfarani Rome

Lucia Ghizzoni Turin

Sandro Loche Cagliari

Mohamad Maghnie Genoa



26 figures, 6 in color and 10 tables, 2016

KARGER Basel · Freiburg · Paris · London · New York · Chennai · New Delhi · Bangkok · Beijing · Shanghai · Tokyo · Kuala Lumpur · Singapore · Sydney

**Endocrine Development**
Founded 1999 by Martin O. Savage, London

**Marco Cappa**
Endocrinology and Diabetology in
Diabetes Units
D.P.U.O.
Bambino Gesù Children's Hospital
IRCCS
Rome, Italy

**Stefano Cianfarani**
Molecular Endocrinology Unit
D.P.U.O.
Bambino Gesù Children's Hospital
IRCCS
'Tor Vergata' University
Rome, Italy

**Lucia Ghizzoni**
Division of Endocrinology, Diabetology and
Metabolism
Department of Internal Medicine
University of Turin
Turin, Italy

**Sandro Loche**
Regional Hospital for Microcytaemia
Cagliari, Italy

**Mohamad Maghnie**
Department of Pediatrics
IRCCS G. Gaslini
University of Genoa
Genoa, Italy

Library of Congress Cataloging-in-Publication Data

Advanced therapies in pediatric endocrinology and diabetology : workshop, Rome, October 27-28, 2014 / volume editors Marco Cappa, Stefano Cianfarani, Lucia Ghizzoni, Sandro Loche, Mohamad Maghnie.
p. ; cm. -- (Endocrine development ; vol. 30)
Includes bibliographical references and index.
ISBN 978-3-318-05636-5 (hard cover : alk. paper) -- ISBN 978-3-318-05637-2 (electronic version)
I. Cappa, Marco, editor. II. Cianfarani, Stefano, editor. III. Ghizzoni, Lucia, editor. IV. Loche, Sandro, editor. V. Maghnie, Mohamad, editor. VI.
Series: Endocrine development ; v. 30.
[DNLM: 1. Endocrine System Diseases--therapy--Congresses. 2. Child--Congresses.
W1 EN3635 v.30 2016 / WS 330]
RJ418
618.92'4--dc23

2015035218

Bibliographic Indices. This publication is listed in bibliographic services, including Current Contents® and PubMed/MEDLINE.

Disclaimer. The statements, opinions and data contained in this publication are solely those of the individual authors and contributors and not of the publisher and the editor(s). The appearance of advertisements in the book is not a warranty, endorsement, or approval of the products or services advertised or of their effectiveness, quality or safety. The publisher and the editor(s) disclaim responsibility for any injury to persons or property resulting from any ideas, methods, instructions or products referred to in the content or advertisements.

Drug Dosage. The authors and the publisher have exerted every effort to ensure that drug selection and dosage set forth in this text are in accord with current recommendations and practice at the time of publication. However, in view of ongoing research, changes in government regulations, and the constant flow of information relating to drug therapy and drug reactions, the reader is urged to check the package insert for each drug for any change in indications and dosage and for added warnings and precautions. This is particularly important when the recommended agent is a new and/or infrequently employed drug.


www.karger.com
Printed in Germany on acid-free and non-aging paper (ISO 9706) by Kraft Druck, Ettlingen
ISSN 1421–7082
e-ISSN 1662–2979
ISBN 978–3–318–05636–5
e-ISBN 978–3–318–05637–2

# Contents

# Preface

This volume of *Endocrine Development* is the 6th volume of a series started in 2007 with the proceedings of an outstanding symposium held in Genoa on congenital endocrinopathies, which was followed by documentations of workshops every other year in different Italian cities (Rome, Cagliari and Turin). The aim of the workshops is to provide an update on advanced therapies of endocrine disorders.

The program of this workshop covered several topics organized in thematic sessions and plenary lectures. Outstanding experts discussed a number of issues, including new modalities for treating type 1 diabetes like the artificial pancreas and islet transplantation in pediatric patients, novel therapeutic approaches for obesity and the metabolic syndrome, as well as adrenal and gonadal disorders.

Recent advances in growth-promoting therapies, such as the C-type natriuretic peptide analogue to treat achondroplasia as well as oxidative stress blockers and gene therapy for patients with adrenoleukodystrophy, have been discussed. The chapters presented are the results of fruitful exchange of scientific information and discussions of experts in the field and we are really grateful to all the participating speakers and authors for sharing their experience and knowledge with us.

We are sure that the quality of this book will be as excellent as the workshop.

*Marco Cappa*, Rome
*Stefano Cianfarani*, Rome
*Lucia Ghizzoni*, Turin
*Sandro Loche*, Cagliari
*Mohamad Maghnie*, Genoa

Cappa M, Cianfarani S, Ghizzoni L, Loche S, Maghnie M (eds): Advanced Therapies in Pediatric Endocrinology and Diabetology. Endocr Dev. Basel, Karger, 2016, vol 30, pp 1–13 (DOI: 10.1159/000439321)

# Toward Automation of Insulin Delivery – Management Solutions for Type 1 Diabetes

Revital Nimri[a] • Moshe Phillip[a, b]

[a]The Jesse Z and Sara Lea Shafer Institute for Endocrinology and Diabetes, National Center for Childhood Diabetes, Schneider Children's Medical Center of Israel, Petah Tikva, and [b]Sackler Faculty of Medicine, Tel Aviv University, Tel Aviv, Israel

**Abstract**

In the past decade, the field of type 1 diabetes was characterized by the efforts to integrate technology into the daily management of diabetes. Automated insulin delivery systems have emerged followed by the improvements in technology of pumps and sensors and automated close-loop systems that were developed around the world for overnight as well as for day and night use. Initially, these closed-loop systems were tested clinically in research centers, then at diabetes camps or hotels, and recently at patients' homes. The systems were tested in a wide range of populations of patients with type 1 diabetes: children, adolescents, adults, newly diagnosed, well and suboptimally controlled patients, the critically ill and pregnant women. The extensive clinical evaluation found these close-loop systems to be safe and efficient in controlling blood glucose levels. Now is the time to take these systems from research to industry and to get a regulatory approval of convenient devices for the use at home. Automated insulin delivery systems have the potential to change the way diabetes is treated and managed for the benefit of patients. This chapter summarizes the recent advances in this field.



A century passed since the discovery of insulin in Toronto and two decades since the results of the Diabetes Control and Complications Trial were published and the world acknowledgment that good glycemic control is mandatory to reduce or postpone diabetes-related complications. In the past years, new technologies have emerged for better blood glucose monitoring, insulin delivery devices, bolus calculators, insulin analogs and more. However, patients and caregivers still struggle to manage diabetes, and the majority of patients with type 1 diabetes around the world do not achieve the desired glycemic control. The data from the pediatric T1D

Exchange clinic registry, which includes 13,316 patients, showed that only 32 and 25% of the patients met the age-specific hemoglobin A1c target levels recommended by the American Diabetes Association and International Society for Pediatric and Adolescent Diabetes, respectively [1]. Maintaining tight glycemic control is associated with an increased risk of hypoglycemia and entails great effort, tension and anxiety that patients with diabetes face at all times. Automated decision support systems and ultimately fully automated management solutions for patients with type 1 diabetes are needed.

The automation of insulin delivery and closed-loop systems have gained the focus of research in diabetes in recent years [2]. The basic principle of these systems is an automated insulin delivery derived by control algorithm which calculates the amount of insulin needed to keep the blood glucose levels within a desired range based on real-time glucose levels measured by a glucose sensor and then delivered automatically to the patient via an insulin pump.

The foundation of the closed-loop approach was laid over 45 years ago by Kadish [3] in 1963. The pioneer system had a real-time continuous glucose monitor and two delivery arms: one for insulin and a counterregulatory arm for glucose or glucagon. However, the system worked on a simple feedback controller and lacked meaningful computer powering. A decade passed until computer control devices were incorporated in the system, creating the 'true artificial pancreas' in 1974 by Albisser et al. [4] in Toronto and Pfeiffer et al. [5] in Germany. The commercial device named Biostator was produced in the 1970s. However, it was a huge and bulky bedside device which needed constant supervision, and hence was abandoned from clinical use. The field of closed-loop insulin delivery was then halted for about two decades. With the remarkable technological progress, including miniaturizations of devices, pumps, interstitial sensors, powered computers and wireless communications, interest in the closed-loop insulin delivery was revived.

Several groups around the world have developed and tested the system in a growing number of clinical studies. These systems were found to be safe, improved metabolic control and solved frequent problems in diabetology. Most importantly, these systems were shown to improve the quality of life of patients and to relieve some of the heavy burden of managing diabetes. The next step is to transfer the software from the clinical research into an industrial product. Based on the results of the clinical trials, it is clear that the time is right for regulatory approval and commercialization of such systems.

## Types of Closed-Loop Systems

A wide range of closed-loop systems have been developed and tested by different research groups around the world. There are two main approaches to automatically control blood glucose excursions in subjects with diabetes. The first and most common approach is the single-hormone delivery of insulin to lower blood glucose. The second is a dual-hormonal delivery approach that adds glucagon as a counter-regulatory hormone together with insulin. Closed-loop systems may also differ in the route for hormone delivery and glucose sensing, and in the type of the control algorithm used.

There are several combinations to monitor glucose levels and deliver insulin in a closed-loop system. The most common closed-loop systems are based on subcutaneous glucose sensing and insulin delivery. This is the most convenient, noninvasive way to close the loop since it is the regular route for insulin delivery and glucose monitoring used nowadays by patients. This kind of closed-loop systems can be more readily approved by regulatory bodies for clinical use since they utilize already available insulin pumps and glucose sensors.

Nevertheless, the use of subcutaneous insulin delivery has several limitations. These include a delay in subcutaneous insulin absorption and action and lack of reproducibility which lead to postprandial hyperglycemia and late hypoglycemia, especially when used to cover meals. These limitations turn the mission of closing the loop during meals into a challenging one. Therefore, another option for closed-loop operation is to sense glucose in the subcutaneous tissue and to deliver insulin intraperitoneally or intravenously in order to improve the insulin action profile and to better mimic the physiological way of insulin delivery.

Renard et al. [6] used an intraperitoneally implanted pump and subcutaneous insulin delivery during closed-loop control for 2 days in 8 adults. However, this method did not overcome the postprandial glucose excursion and patients still needed to give a preprandial insulin bolus. The disadvantages of this approach include the need to implant a pump and to periodically refill it with insulin in the hospital, risk of site infection and increased risk to develop insulin antibodies.

Different types of control algorithms were developed over the past years. These sophisticated calculators utilize transmitted glucose levels for analysis of the needed insulin treatment dose. In addition, several systems set individualized target glucose levels and take the diversity in insulin sensitivity in different patients and within the same patient into consideration. Thus, a closed-loop system needs to be personalized and to have an active and dynamic system that can change treatment periodically according to real-time learning of the unpredictable behavior of glucose-insulin dynamics [7].

The first control algorithm that was used clinically was the proportional-integral-derivative algorithm by Steil et al. [8]. Their control algorithm had three components that all together dictated the amount of the total insulin treatment dose: the proportional component calculated the deviation of the blood glucose level from the target glucose level, the integral component calculated the area under the curve between the blood and target glucose level, and the third derivative component took into account the rate of glucose change into account. There is another way to calculate the needed amount of insulin which is by using of the model predictive controller (MPC). This

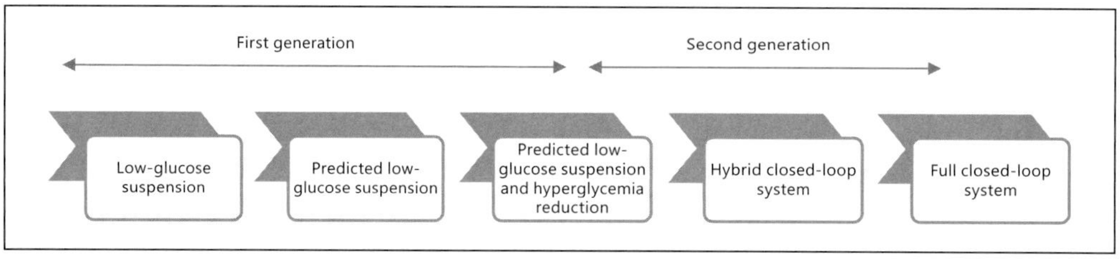


**Fig. 1.** Artificial pancreas step/generation diagram – the development pathway (with permission from JDRF).

control algorithm – which is mostly used and studied – predicts the upcoming blood glucose levels based on physiological models of human glucose metabolism. The algorithm adjusts the insulin treatment in order to bring the predicted glucose levels into the target range. These two types of algorithms use mathematical models to link glucose excursions to insulin demands.

An alternative way to calculate insulin delivery is to use the regular set of rules that patients and caregivers use to treat and manage diabetes in daily life. This method of insulin delivery is a unique clinical-driven technology based on a fuzzy logic control algorithm [9].

### The Pathway Towards Closed-Loop Systems

Closed-loop systems were recognized by several important organizations as a potential management solution for patients with type 1 diabetes. In 2006, the Juvenile Diabetes Research Foundation (JDRF) and in 2010 the European Union established the artificial pancreas consortiums (JDRF Artificial Pancreas Project and AP@Home). These organizations and others have been making great efforts to promote the development of a commercially available artificial pancreas.

The JDRF strategic for stepwise implementation of automated insulin delivery is presented in the – 'artificial pancreas step/generation' diagram (fig. 1). This strategy includes three generations of automated insulin delivery systems. The first generation includes the devices that shut off insulin delivery to prevent episodes of hypoglycemia. Hypoglycemia remains a major barrier for glycemic control even in the era of advanced technologies. The second generation consists of closed-loop systems that are able to increase the time within the target range and reduce the rate of hypoglycemia. This category includes two closed-loop systems: one system that allows a certain degree of patient involvement at meal or physical activity announcement (hybrid closed-loop system) and the other is the ultimate desired system with no need from the patient to intervene (full closed-loop system). As delineated by the JDRF, the third generation includes the future device for closed-loop systems that will incorporate other hormones besides insulin.

### Low/Predicted Glucose Suspension

The first generation of automated insulin delivery devices is featured with the aim to reduce hypoglycemia. These technologies include the low and predicted glucose suspension features incorporated in the sensor-augmented pump therapy.

The first approved automated insulin delivery system is the threshold-suspend feature of the sensor-augmented insulin pumps (MiniMed 530G System; Medtronic Diabetes, Northridge, Calif., USA). This feature is designed to automatically suspend insulin delivery for up to 2 h when the glucose level reaches a predefined low sensor glucose threshold [10].

The safety and efficacy of this system in reducing the risk of nocturnal hypoglycemia was tested in several clinical studies by the ASPIRE In-Home study group. Two large-scale studies point out the efficacy of this system in reducing hypoglycemia with a mild but nonsignificant increase in hyperglycemia [11, 12].

Bergenstal et al. [11] studied 247 subjects with type 1 diabetes prone to nocturnal hypoglycemia treated with insulin pump therapy. Subjects were randomly assigned to participate in a 3-month study with or without the threshold-suspend feature activated in their pumps. The glucose threshold for insulin suspension was 70 mg/dl. After 3 months, the mean area under the curve of 65 mg/dl for nocturnal hypoglycemic events was 37.5% lower in the group who used the low-glucose suspend (LGS) feature compared to the control group. Thus, the use of the LGS feature reduces the risk of nocturnal hypoglycemia when it occurs as expected. But, unpredictably, it also showed a 31.8% reduction in the frequency of nocturnal hypoglycemia. This observation was speculated to be related to improved counterregulatory hormone responses as a consequence of a shorter duration of hypoglycemia events, and therefore minimized hypoglycemia-associated autonomic failure. The reduction in the hypoglycemia risk was found to be safe and was not associated with an increase in glycated hemoglobin values or significant reactive postsuspension hyperglycemia [11]. The LGS feature was also found to reduce the risk of overall severe and moderate hypoglycemia in a randomized controlled study involving 95 patients in a 6-month intervention period [12].

The advantage of the LGS feature was demonstrated in a retrospective analysis of data from 20,973 patients who used this feature on a regular basis. Results showed that on days on which the LGS feature was activated, patients experienced 69% fewer hypoglycemic episodes below 50 mg/dl compared to days on which the feature was not activated. The effect was more prominent overnight than during daytime [13].

The next step in automation of insulin delivery is to suspend insulin delivery before hypoglycemia occurs, in response to a predicted predefined low sensor value. Buckingham et al. [14, 15] conducted feasibility studies in ambulatory and patients' home settings. The results of these studies showed a reduction in hypoglycemia with a slight increase in mean overnight glucose levels. In another feasibility study, Danne et al. [16] tested the ability of the predicted LGS (PLGS) to reduce the occurrence of exercise-induced hypoglycemia. The results of this study imply that this system prevents hypoglycemia by suspending insulin about half an hour before a predicted hypoglycemic event. Recently, Maahs et al. [17] tested the PLGS only for the nighttime in 45 subjects for 42 nights with and without the PLGS. The median area under the curve of 60 mg/dl for nocturnal hypoglycemic events was 81% lower in the group who used the PLGS feature than for the control group. Nevertheless, the reduction in hypoglycemia was associated with significantly higher mean overnight and morning glucose levels. More studies are needed in order to demonstrate that the use of PLGS indeed reduces the risk of hypoglycemia without jeopardizing the glycemic control.

In summary, LGS and PLGS technologies showed the ability to reduce the rate of hypoglycemia but with mild elevation of blood glucose levels since these technologies are unable to adjust insulin for the hyperglycemic range, as compared to hybrid or full closed-loop systems.

The next-generation device in this group may include, in addition to the PLGS, also an automated administration of insulin bolus when the blood glucose reaches a predefined hyperglycemia threshold, thus advancing in a stepwise approach to a full closed-loop system.

## Clinical Studies of Closed-Loop Systems

The second generation of automated insulin delivery is the closed-loop systems, which have a real-time feedback control on blood glucose levels. These systems have currently two operation modes: (a) the hybrid closed-loop system – an automated closed-loop system which allows manual insulin delivery by the patient, such as an insulin bolus before meals, and (b) the full closed-loop system – all insulin is automatically delivered by the system.

One of the most challenging tasks of diabetes management in general and closed-loop control in particular is to identify the glycemic effects of the food consumed. The use of different closed-loop controllers cannot completely eliminate the frequently found postprandial glucose excursions above the target range. This happens mainly due to a delay in subcutaneous insulin absorption and action. It also takes about 20 min [9] to detect a meal event and react with a bolus of insulin that takes about 1 h to reduce postprandial hyperglycemia. A more aggressive insulin treatment for meals might reduce postprandial hyperglycemia but, on the other hand, may cause postprandial hypoglycemia. Hence, most current closed-loop systems use the approach of hybrid closed-loop control [2]. Therefore, meal treatment is currently handled in most closed-loop systems by a manual bolus before the meal given by the patients. Different types of boluses before a meal are used in different closed-loop systems, including 25–100% of the calculated manual bolus or a small amount of priming insulin given before a meal and the rest automatically by the closed-loop system. Another way to calculate the amount of priming insulin is done as the patient announces the type of the meal (breakfast, lunch or dinner) and the size of the meal.

The next step in the development of closed-loop systems is to overcome the meal challenge and to have a full closed-loop system where the patient does not need to give any input to the system. Several other attempts to improve postprandial glucose excretions include the use of glucagon suppressors: pramlintide (amylin analog) or exenatide (glucagon-like peptide-1 analog) with limited effect on postprandial blood glucose levels during closed-loop control [18, 19]. Another method is the attempt to accelerate insulin absorption and action by local warming of the insulin infusion site and thus improving postprandial glucose excursions [20]. All the current endeavors have not yet shown any significant advantage over insulin treatment alone. The possibility of full closed-loop control may be feasible when new and faster insulin will be available.

## Overnight Closed-Loop Systems

The barrier in treating meals led some groups to focus on automated control of blood glucose during the night as it is 'not complicated by meals' most of the time. Other important reasons to concentrate on the nighttime were the need to reduce the risk of nocturnal hypoglycemia, to improve overnight control as patients cannot react to their blood glucose levels while sleeping, and to improve morning blood glucose, since lower morning glucose levels were found to have a positive effect on glucose control during the day.

Nocturnal hypoglycemia is a common and worrying occurrence in type 1 diabetes. Nocturnal hypoglycemia is hard to predict and can occur to any patient even the poorly controlled patients with elevated blood glucose most of the time. Most of the severe and life-threatening hypoglycemic events occur at night even when patients use a glucose sensor [21]. In addition, nonsevere hypoglycemic events were found to impair mood and well-being, memory consolidation and sleep quality, and to increase physical fatigue on the subsequent day [22]. Therefore, overnight glycemic control and prevention of nocturnal hypoglycemia are unmet needs that can be treated with overnight closed-loop control.

Several groups tested extensively closed-loop systems during overnight use. The group from Cambridge [23–25] using the MPC algorithm, the Florence system and the DREAM (Diabetes Wireless Artificial Pancreas Consortium) group [26–28] using fuzzy logic controller – the MD-Logic system. Other groups tested their closed-loop system for an overnight period in small studies: the Medtronic group [29] and the Virginia group [30].

DREAM is a partnership group from centers in Slovenia, Germany and Israel. The aim of the group is to promote the recognition of the MD-Logic closed-loop system as a tool to control overnight blood glucose and reduce nocturnal hypoglycemia. The

DREAM group conducted inpatient [31, 32], transitional [27] and more substantial home studies [26, 28, 33]. These studies showed that the MD-Logic system is safe for home use and effective in reducing the occurrence, duration and severity of hypoglycemia while improving overnight metabolic control. This system was the first to be used at patients' homes in 2012. Since then the system has been evaluated in several home studies, each time for a longer duration: 4 nights, 6 weeks and recently 3 months of overnight use. In all studies, the use of the system demonstrated improvement in glycemic control and reduced hypoglycemia over sensor-augmented pump therapy. The 4-night study included 75 children, adolescents and adults from the three DREAM diabetes consortium centers who participated in a crossover, single-blind study. Interim analysis showed that the time which glucose levels were below 70 mg/dl was significantly shorter on the closed-loop nights than on control nights with medians (interquartile ranges) of 3.8 (0–11.6) and 48.7 min (0.6–67.9), respectively ($p = 0.0034$), and that the time within the desired range of 70–140 mg/dl was significantly increased, with a similar amount of insulin in the two arms [26, 34]. The results of the entire study of the 75 patients were similar [34].

The next study tested the system in 24 subjects for 6 weeks overnight compared to sensor-augmented pump therapy at patients' homes during regular daily life [28]. Time spent in hypoglycemia was significantly reduced ($p = 0.02$) and the percentage of time spent at the target range was increased ($p = 0.003$). Interestingly, this improvement was achieved with a lower amount of insulin, and, moreover, the improved morning glucose levels achieved by the MD-Logic system were found to have a positive effect on daytime glycemic control.

A pooled analysis of these two studies showed that the improved overnight glucose control under the MD-Logic system was seen irrespective of baseline hemoglobin A1c, age or gender. Therefore, this technology should work for every patient with diabetes.

The group from Cambridge also conducted inpatient overnight studies with their MPC algorithm [23]. This group also tested the closed loop at patients' homes: a pediatric study lasting 3 weeks [35] and an adult study lasting 4 weeks [36]. The pooled analysis [25] of these results, covering 40 subjects, showed an increase in the time spent within the range of 70–144 mg/dl (by a median of 18.5%), an improvement achieved by a greater amount of insulin given overnight, with a similar rate of hypoglycemia for the adults [36] and the pediatric group [35].

### Day and Night Closed-Loop Systems

The ultimate goal of closed-loop systems is the development of a commercially available automated insulin delivery system for the management of type 1 diabetes. This system can change the way diabetes is treated and managed by using full 24-hour closed-loop control in the daily routine of the patients. Daytime glycemic control is challenging primarily because it is 'complicated' by meals and physical activity, as was already mentioned.

The first attempt to use a closed-loop system to control blood glucose levels was during the day and night and was done by Steil et al. [8] in 2006. This system was based on a proportional-integral-derivative algorithm and was tested in 10 adults. This study provided a proof of concept that glycemic control can be achieved with fully automated insulin delivery. From that point on, several groups tested closed-loop systems for day and night use. Most of the studies were conducted in hospital-protected environment and included small numbers of patients for 24–60 h of closed-loop control. The group from Cambridge tested 12 adolescents for 36-hour with hybrid closed-loop control (including meals and exercise). The percentage of time within the target range (70–180 mg/dl) was significantly improved during closed-loop control compared to pump therapy alone during 24 h [median (IQR) 74 (69–79) compared to 47 (25–54)] without a difference for the daytime [55 (48–71) and 49 (47–71), respectively] [37]. A similar study by the same group evaluated closed-loop control for 26 h in a group of very young subjects, aged 2–7 years, compared to pump therapy alone. Glycemic control was similar between the two groups, the only advantage of closed-loop control being the reduction in nighttime hyperglycemia above 300 mg/dl (0.18 vs. 1.3 h, $p = 0.035$) [38]. These studies showed that most of the impact of this closed-loop system was attributed to the nighttime control and not to daytime benefits.

The different study methodologies and the way data were analyzed make it difficult to compare the performance of different closed-loop algorithms. In an interesting multicenter, multinational in-hospital study, two MPC algorithms were tested in hybrid mode (the Cambridge and the International Artificial Pancreas groups) in comparison to conventional insulin pump treatment for 24 h (48 adult participants). Hypoglycemia was reduced with both algorithms, but the reduction in hypoglycemia was accompanied with greater hyperglycemia and elevation of mean blood glucose levels when compared to treatment with insulin pump therapy alone [39]. Several studies tested the closed-loop system for day and night use outside the hospital environment. The first feasibility study was conducted by the AP@Home consortium where 17 adults used closed-loop control for 1 week and insulin pump therapy for another week in a randomized order at patients' homes. The time within the target range increased by 13% with no change in time spent in hypoglycemia. The 24-hour improvement was attributed mainly to the nighttime improvement, which is easier to achieve compared to daytime alone [40].

The DREAM consortium evaluated 60 h of closed-loop control with the MD-Logic system over the weekend in 22 children, adolescents and adults. MD-Logic control increased the time within the range and decreased median glucose levels during closed-loop control compared to sensor-augmented pump therapy with a comparable low rate of hypoglycemia in both groups. The improved glycemic control observed during MD-Logic use was accomplished with an insulin dose similar to that used in the control arm. These findings might be related to both the improved timing and dosage of the insulin delivery and the system dosing method of combined basal and bolus administration, which favor the way of treatment rather than the overall integrative insulin dosage [33].

Several small studies tested the bihormonal closed-loop approach during day and night control. Russell et al. [41] reported results of two similar studies testing a bihormonal closed-loop system for 5 days. Twenty adults used the closed-loop system at a hotel environment and compared the results to home use of insulin pump treatment. Thirty-two adolescents used the system at a diabetes camp compared to insulin pump therapy. The control group did not necessarily use continuous glucose monitoring. Data were analyzed excluding the 1st day and showed a decrease in mean blood glucose levels in adults and adolescents with a reduction in time in hypoglycemia for the adult group and no change in hypoglycemia in the adolescent group between closed-loop control and insulin pump therapy [41].

Another study at home tested the bihormonal algorithm for 48 h in 11 adult patients. Results showed that the time spent in the target range was comparable and median glucose levels were lower on the 2nd day at the expense of more time in hypoglycemia between closed- and open-loop control [42].

Although closed-loop studies with different algorithms have different methodologies and structures, the data on the performance of the bihormonal system seem similar to systems that use a single hormone (insulin). Nevertheless, this approach raises concerns about glucagon stability and effectiveness over time, with the possibility that glucagon would not be constant in counteracting the overdelivery of insulin and thus may occasionally cause hypoglycemia.

A remarkable advancement has been made in the last decade toward automation of insulin delivery for patients with type 1 diabetes. The advancement in insulin pump devices and especially better glucose sensors with improved accuracy have led to nearby available automated insulin delivery systems to manage diabetes for regular use. A diversity of closed-loop systems was tested in a growing number of patients and recently at patients' homes for overnight and day and night use. These studies show that closed-loop systems enable a better glycemic control, increase the time within the range with no change or even a reduction in the occurrence of hypoglycemia. This technological 'cure' for diabetes will be a bridge until a biological cure will, hopefully, be found.

## Psychological Effects of Closed-Loop Control

Few studies addressed the psychological aspects and acceptance of closed-loop system use at home. Ziegler et al. [43] assessed the impact of overnight use of the MD-Logic system at home regarding fear of hypoglycemia, satisfaction and acceptance of the new technology among children, adolescents and adults. Worries concerning episodes of hypoglycemia were significantly reduced when using the MD-Logic system compared to sensor-augmented pump therapy (p = 0.017). Perceived ease of use as a determinant of acceptance with the closed-loop system significantly increased (p = 0.002). The overall satisfaction mean score after intervention was 3.02 ± 0.54 (range 0–4), demonstrating a high level of satisfaction with the system [43]. Satisfaction from closed-loop overnight use at home was also reported by the Cambridge group among adult participants [44]. Data were collected from 24 patients' interviews. Most patients mentioned the following positive key themes: improved blood glucose control, reassurance/reduced worry, improved overnight control leading to improved daily functioning and diabetes control. The key negative themes were: technical difficulties and intrusiveness of alarms. Of the 24 participants, 20 would recommend the closed-loop technology.

Nevertheless, closed-loop systems have their limitations. These systems can do the best out of the existing device components of the closed loop: pump, sensor and the current insulin. The sensor which is the heart of the system has several limitations mainly concerning accuracy and reliability, which is crucial for closed-loop operation. Therefore, reliable systems need to have sufficient risk mitigations for situations of sensor inaccuracy, sensor artifact, drifts, sensor pullout and disrupted communication with the sensor. Patients still need to wear a sensor that depends on manual calibrations and need to invest efforts to operate the sensor. The pump also has limitations that have an impact on the closed-loop operation, especially pump occlusions. And, undoubtedly, a 'faster' insulin, with rapid absorption and action profile will have a major impact on closed-loop performance, and improve postprandial glucose excursions, thus, enabling a full closed-loop operation.

In summary, closed-loop systems were found to be safe. They add value as a means of metabolic control for any given patient, they are associated with better control and reduced risk of hypoglycemia, they are accurate enough for clinical use, they solve frequent problems in diabetology and, most importantly for patients, they improve quality of life and relieve some of the heavy burden of managing diabetes.

## References


1 Wood JR, Miller KM, Maahs DM, et al: Most youth with type 1 diabetes in the T1D Exchange Clinic Registry do not meet American Diabetes Association or International Society for Pediatric and Adolescent Diabetes clinical guidelines. Diabetes Care 2013;36:2035–2037.

2 Nimri R, Phillip M: Artificial pancreas: fuzzy logic and control of glycemia. Curr Opin Endocrinol Diabetes Obes 2014;21:251–256.

3 Kadish A: Automation control of blood sugar: a servomechanism for glucose monitoring and control. Trans Am Soc Artif Intern Organs 1963;9:363–367.

4 Albisser AM, Leibel BS, Ewart TG, et al: Clinical control of diabetes by the artificial pancreas. Diabetes 1974;23:397–404.

5 Pfeiffer E, Thum C, Clemens A: The artificial beta cell – a continuous control of blood sugar by external regulation of insulin infusion (glucose controlled insulin infusion system). Horm Metab Res 1974;6:339–342.

6 Renard E, Place J, Cantwell M, Chevassus H, Palerm CC: Closed-loop insulin delivery using a subcutaneous glucose sensor and intraperitoneal insulin delivery: feasibility study testing a new model for the artificial pancreas. Diabetes Care 2010;33:121–127.

7 Miller S, Nimri R, Atlas E, Grunberg EA, Phillip M: Automatic learning algorithm for the MD-Logic artificial pancreas system. Diabetes Technol Ther 2011;13:983–990.
8 Steil G, Rebrin K, Darwin C, Hariri F, Saad M: Feasibility of automating insulin delivery for the treatment of type 1 diabetes. Diabetes 2006;55:3344–3350.
9 Atlas E, Nimri R, Miller S, Grunberg E, Phillip M: MD-Logic artificial pancreas system: a pilot study in adults with type 1 diabetes. Diabetes Care 2010;33: 1072–1076.
10 Pickup JC: Semi-closed-loop insulin delivery systems: early experience with low-glucose insulin suspend pumps. Diabetes Technol Ther 2011;13:695–698.
11 Bergenstal RM, Klonoff DC, Garg SK, et al: Threshold-based insulin-pump interruption for reduction of hypoglycemia. N Engl J Med 2013;369:224–232.
12 Ly TT, Nicholas JA, Retterath A, Lim EM, Davis EA, Jones TW: Effect of sensor-augmented insulin pump therapy and automated insulin suspension vs standard insulin pump therapy on hypoglycemia in patients with type 1 diabetes: a randomized clinical trial. JAMA 2013;310:1240–1247.
13 Agrawal P, Zhong A, Welsh JB, Shah R, Kaufman FR: Retrospective analysis of the real-world use of the threshold suspend feature of sensor-augmented insulin pumps. Diabetes Technol Ther 2015;17:316–319.
14 Buckingham B, Cobry E, Clinton P, et al: Preventing hypoglycemia using predictive alarm algorithms and insulin pump suspension. Diabetes Technol Ther 2009;11:93–97.
15 Buckingham BA, Cameron F, Calhoun P, et al: Outpatient safety assessment of an in-home predictive low-glucose suspend system with type 1 diabetes subjects at elevated risk of nocturnal hypoglycemia. Diabetes Technol Ther 2013;15:622–627.
16 Danne T, Tsioli C, Kordonouri O, et al: The PILGRIM study: in silico modeling of a predictive low glucose management system and feasibility in youth with type 1 diabetes during exercise. Diabetes Technol Ther 2014;16:338–347.
17 Maahs DM, Calhoun P, Buckingham BA, et al: A randomized trial of a home system to reduce nocturnal hypoglycemia in type 1 diabetes. Diabetes Care 2014;37:1885–1891.
18 Renukuntla VS, Ramchandani N, Trast J, Cantwell M, Heptulla RA: Role of glucagon-like peptide-1 analogue versus amylin as an adjuvant therapy in type 1 diabetes in a closed loop setting with ePID algorithm. J Diabetes Sci Technol 2014;8:1011–1017.
19 Weinzimer SA, Sherr JL, Cengiz E, et al: Effect of pramlintide on prandial glycemic excursions during closed-loop control in adolescents and young adults with type 1 diabetes. Diabetes Care 2012;35:1994–1999.
20 Freckmann G, Pleus S, Haug C, Bitton G, Nagar R: Increasing local blood flow by warming the application site: beneficial effects on postprandial glycemic excursions. J Diabetes Sci Technol 2012;6:780–785.
21 Buckingham B, Block J, Burdick J, et al: Response to nocturnal alarms using a real-time glucose sensor. Diabetes Technol Ther 2005;7:440–447.
22 King P, Kong MF, Parkin H, Macdonald IA, Tattersall RB: Well-being, cerebral function, and physical fatigue after nocturnal hypoglycemia in IDDM. Diabetes Care 1998;21:341–345.
23 Hovorka R, Allen J, Elleri D, et al: Manual closed-loop insulin delivery in children and adolescents with type 1 diabetes: a phase 2 randomised crossover trial. Lancet 2010;375:743–751.
24 Elleri D, Allen JM, Nodale M, et al: Automated overnight closed-loop glucose control in young children with type 1 diabetes. Diabetes Technol Ther 2011;13: 419–424.
25 Thabit H, Elleri D, Leelarathna L, et al: Unsupervised home use of overnight closed-loop system over 3–4 weeks: a pooled analysis of randomized controlled studies in adults and adolescents with type 1 diabetes. Diabetes Obes Metab 2015;17:452–458.
26 Nimri R, Muller I, Atlas E, et al: Night glucose control with MD-Logic artificial pancreas in home setting: a single blind, randomized crossover trial-interim analysis. Pediatr Diabetes 2014;15:91–99.
27 Phillip M, Battelino T, Atlas E, et al: Nocturnal glucose control with an artificial pancreas at a diabetes camp. N Engl J Med 2013;368:824–833.
28 Nimri R, Muller I, Atlas E, et al: MD-Logic overnight control for 6 weeks of home use in patients with type 1 diabetes: randomized crossover trial. Diabetes Care 2014;37:3025–3032.
29 O'Grady MJ, Retterath AJ, Keenan DB, et al: The use of an automated, portable glucose control system for overnight glucose control in adolescents and young adults with type 1 diabetes. Diabetes Care 2012;35: 2182–2187.
30 Clarke W, Anderson S, Breton M, Patek S, Kashmer L, Kovatchev B: Closed-loop artificial pancreas using subcutaneous glucose sensing and insulin delivery and a model predictive control algorithm: the Virginia experience. J Diabetes Sci Technol 2009;3: 1031–1038.
31 Nimri R, Atlas E, Ajzensztejn M, Miller S, Oron T, Phillip M: Feasibility study of automated overnight closed-loop glucose control under MD-Logic artificial pancreas in patients with type 1 diabetes: the DREAM Project. Diabetes Technol Ther 2012;14: 728–735.
32 Nimri R, Danne T, Kordonouri O, et al: The 'Glucositter' overnight automated closed loop system for type 1 diabetes: a randomized crossover trial. Pediatr Diabetes 2013;14:159–167.

33 Nimri R, DREAM Consortium: Integration of the MD-Logic into daily management of diabetes. 8th International Conference on Advanced Technologies and Treatments for Diabetes, Paris, 2015.
34 Danne T, Muller I: An overnight automated closed-loop, MD-Logic system at patient's home. 7th International Conference on Advanced Technologies and Treatments for Diabetes, Vienna, 2014.
35 Hovorka R, Elleri D, Thabit H, et al: Overnight closed-loop insulin delivery in young people with type 1 diabetes: a free-living, randomized clinical trial. Diabetes Care 2014;37:1204–1211.
36 Thabit H, Lubina-Solomon A, Stadler M, et al: Home use of closed-loop insulin delivery for overnight glucose control in adults with type 1 diabetes: a 4-week, multicentre, randomised crossover study. Lancet Diabetes Endocrinol 2014;2:701–709.
37 Elleri D, Allen JM, Kumareswaran K, et al: Closed-loop basal insulin delivery over 36 h in adolescents with type 1 diabetes: randomized clinical trial. Diabetes Care 2013;36:838–844.
38 Dauber A, Corcia L, Safer J, Agus MS, Einis S, Steil GM: Closed-loop insulin therapy improves glycemic control in children aged <7 years: a randomized controlled trial. Diabetes Care 2013;36:222–227.
39 Luijf YM, DeVries JH, Zwinderman K, et al: Day and night closed-loop control in adults with type 1 diabetes: a comparison of two closed-loop algorithms driving continuous subcutaneous insulin infusion versus patient self-management. Diabetes Care 2013; 36:3882–3887.
40 Leelarathna L, Dellweg S, Mader JK, et al: Day and night home closed-loop insulin delivery in adults with type 1 diabetes: three-center randomized crossover study. Diabetes Care 2014;37:1931–1937.
41 Russell SJ, El-Khatib FH, Sinha M, et al: Outpatient glycemic control with a bionic pancreas in type 1 diabetes. N Engl J Med 2014;371:313–325.
42 van Bon AC, Luijf YM, Koebrugge R, Koops R, Hoekstra JB, Devries JH: Feasibility of a portable bihormonal closed-loop system to control glucose excursions at home under free-living conditions for 48 h. Diabetes Technol Ther 2014;16:131–136.
43 Ziegler C, Liberman A, Nimri R, Müller I, Klemencic S, Bratina N, Bläsig S, Remus K, Phillip M, Battelino T, Kordonouri O, Danne T, Lange K: Reduced worries of hypoglycaemia, high satisfaction and increased perceived ease of use after experiencing four nights of MD-Logic artificial pancreas at home (DREAM 4). J Diabetes Res 2015, http://www.hindawi.com/journals/jdr/aa/590308/cta/.
44 Barnard KD, Wysocki T, Thabit H, et al: Psychosocial aspects of closed- and open-loop insulin delivery: closing the loop in adults with type 1 diabetes in the home setting. Diabet Med 2015;32:601–608.

Moshe Phillip, MD
The Jesse Z and Sara Lea Shafer Institute for Endocrinology and Diabetes
National Center for Childhood Diabetes, Schneider Children's Medical Center of Israel
14 Kaplan Street, Petah Tikva 4920235 (Israel)
E-Mail mosheph@post.tau.ac.il

Cappa M, Cianfarani S, Ghizzoni L, Loche S, Maghnie M (eds): Advanced Therapies in Pediatric Endocrinology and Diabetology. Endocr Dev. Basel, Karger, 2016, vol 30, pp 14–22 (DOI: 10.1159/000439322)

# Islet Transplantation in Pediatric Patients: Current Indications and Future Perspectives

Federico Bertuzzi[a] · Barbara Antonioli[b] · Marta C. Tosca[b] · Marta Galuzzi[b] · Matteo Bonomo[a] · Mario Marazzi[b] · Giacomo Colussi[c]

[a]Diabetology Unit, [b]Tissue Therapy Unit and [c]Nephrology Department, Niguarda Hospital, Milan, Italy

**Abstract**

The first islet transplantation in diabetes mellitus was performed more than 20 years ago. Since then, clinical results have progressively improved. Nowadays, islet transplantation can be considered a real therapeutic option after pancreatectomy for painful chronic pancreatitis (autotransplantation) and in selected adult patients affected by type 1 diabetes mellitus (allotransplantation). Better results are mainly due to the advances in the standardization of islet isolation and purification procedures as well as in the pharmacological treatment of recipients. Anti-inflammatory treatments facilitate islet engraftment and prevent metabolic exhaustion and functional β-cell apoptosis; new strategies better control islet graft rejection. As a consequence, islet transplantation activities are no longer confined to few centers only, rather thousands of transplants are now performed all over the world. Many attempts are actually undertaken to find solutions to current problems of islets transplantation, from toxicity of immunosuppressive therapy to the limited engraftment, function and duration. There is general hope that these procedures will offer a safe and feasible therapeutic option for an increasing number of patients suffering from diabetes mellitus, including pediatric patients.



Today, islet transplantation represents a therapeutic option for selected patients affected by diabetes mellitus under insulin treatment. Although the first islet transplantation was performed more than 20 years ago, there is still great interest in this procedure. Clinical results have progressively improved, and in some centers the rate of insulin independence after islet transplantation is now similar to that of whole pancreas transplantation [1]. Islet transplantation actually remains the only minimally invasive treatment able to restore normoglycemia without exogenous insulin administration in patients affected by type 1 diabetes mellitus.

## Current Clinical Indications of Islet Transplantation in Adults

Islet transplantation is indicated as β-cell replacement in selected cases when β-cell function is completely lost. The main clinical indications in adults are (1) allotransplantation in patients with type 1 diabetes mellitus already under immunosuppressive therapy for another transplantation (kidney and/or liver) or (2) with brittle diabetes characterized by unstable glycemia and acute diabetic complications, and (3) autotransplantation in patients undergoing total pancreatectomy for chronic pancreatitis with intractable pain [2].

Chronic pancreatitis is a benign disease that leads to irreversible and severe damage of both exocrine and endocrine functions. In histological evaluation, it is characterized by fibrosis, duct obstruction and inflammation. The clinical manifestations vary as to the degree of pain (often intractable), impaired digestion, exocrine function loss and the occurrence of diabetes. Intractable pain often requires high doses of narcotics with frequent hospitalizations [3]. Pancreatectomy cures pain but provokes a severe enzyme deficiency and the onset of diabetes, which are difficult to manage. Glycemic control is in fact complex not only with regard to insulin deficiency, but also due to the lack of glucagon production, the hormone that increases blood glucose levels and is secreted to prevent hypoglycemia. Islet transplantation is a possible solution to improve the management of diabetes mellitus following total pancreatectomy [4]. Islets are isolated from the surgically excised pancreas, and after purification of the exocrine component, they are transplanted back into the same patient. The islet isolation procedure is often a difficult challenge due to the chronic inflammatory, fibrotic condition of the organ, which is sometimes calcific and of small volume [5]. In this case, the pancreas presents structural alterations that represent an obstacle to the intraparenchymal spread of lytic enzymes involved in organ digestion. In addition, chronic inflammation damages the exocrine tissue structure and composition, reducing the density difference towards the β cells and thereby preventing their separation by density gradient centrifugation. The result is often the retrieval of a small number of islets which are often not well purified by the exocrine component. Immunosuppression is not required in this specific context of autotransplantation. In addition, patients after pancreatectomy are less insulin resistant and inflammation is less severe, with no risk of autoimmune reactivation compared to the patients with type 1 diabetes mellitus. The final result is that islet engraftment is favored and a lower number of isolated islets are usually required to achieve insulin independence compared to allotransplantation. The number of transplanted islets appears to be the most important determinant of glycemic control in recipients. The minimum number of islets needed to achieve insulin independence has been suggested to vary from 2,000 to 6,000 islet equivalents per kilogram of the recipient's body weight [3–5]. Once insulin independence is reached, progressive functional exhaustion of the endocrine cells may occur in some patients. This phenomenon has been attributed to several causes, mainly the block of regenerative processes in the islets once engrafted in another tissue. It is well known that pancreatic islets, during their life, are subjected to a process of rearrangement with the formation of new β cells probably starting from precursors that accumulating evidence suggests to be intrapancreatic, perhaps of ductal origin. This process is responsible for the adaptation of the function to the variable β-cellular metabolic demand [6]. In islet transplantation, this process is profoundly altered, and in the long term it can lead to a progressive decrease in and exhaustion of β-cell function [7].

After total pancreatectomy and islet transplantation, most patients have less pain and overall a better quality of life. The percentages of patients with insulin independence are variable in relation to the experience of the center and the amount of transplanted islets, but on average they are obtained in 50% of patients (from 30 to 70% in relation to the number of transplanted islets) [3]. Thanks to these positive results, clinical indication of islet autotransplantation has recently expanded and has been extended to the loss of pancreatic parenchyma for the resection of both benign and malignant tumors of the pancreas or after total pancreatectomy for severe abdominal trauma. There are no published reports of pancreatic malignant disease occurring in the liver and related to islet autotransplantation [8]. Therefore, islet autotransplantation can contribute to prevent diabetes even in partial pancreatectomy.

Islet transplantation is also proposed in selected patients with type 1 diabetes mellitus in combined transplantation or in brittle diabetes mellitus in cases where the pancreas transplantation in toto is not possible. These cases include cardiovascular or cerebral diseases or other clinical conditions that contraindicate a major surgery. In addition, in selected cases, patients prefer a more simple intervention under local anesthesia (islet transplantation) to a severe surgical operation. Therefore, clinical indications for islet allotransplantation are: (1) brittle type 1 diabetes mellitus; (2) combined organ transplant (kidney, first of all, but also liver or heart) in type 1 diabetes, and (3) the need for immunosuppressive therapy for other autoimmune diseases in addition to type 1 diabetes.

In patients already on immunosuppressive therapy for autoimmune diseases or organ transplantation, islet transplantation and the subsequent immunosuppressive therapy itself may require minor adaptations or none at all. Instead, in unstable, non-immunosuppressed type 1 diabetes mellitus patients, immunosuppressive therapy is specifically needed for islet transplantation: it is common belief that clinical conditions in these patients have to be severe enough as to justify this choice. For this reason, only selected patients will be potential candidates for islet transplantation, those who were not adequately treated by the standard therapeutic strategies [9].

The definition of unstable diabetes has long been controversial: the glucose variability might be secondary to inadequate patient management/ability or educational training. However, it is well known that even through accurate blood sugar level self-control as well as frequent visits to the diabetologist, a small number of patients suffer serious glycemia instability with sudden and frequent episodes of hypoglycemia or ketoacidosis and very poor overall quality of life. This clinical condition is known as brittle diabetes [9]. The diagnosis excludes the various pathologies or factors that alter glucose homeostasis and blood sugar levels in patients, as well as factitious diabetes and psychological instability. For these patients, therapeutic strategies require the treatment of secondary causes of the brittleness and the optimization of the standard insulin therapy using continuous subcutaneous insulin infusion alone or integrated with continuous glucose monitoring; only finally they should be considered for substitution of β-cell function with isolated pancreas or islet transplantation.

Islet transplantation efficacy can be assessed in terms of insulin dose variation, reduction in acute and chronic complications, hypoglycemia episodes and the overall quality of life impact. In the whole, all these clinical parameters have generally improved together with the number of islet transplantations in the past years.

According to the Collaborative Islet Transplant Registry that collects data on clinical islet isolations and transplants, islet retrieval has improved over time as well as the number of transplanted islets per recipient. Similarly, the insulin independence rate has progressively improved: 3 years after transplant it increased from 27% in 1999–2002 to 37% in 2003–2006 and to 44% in 2007–2010. C-peptide ≥0.3 ng/ml, which is indicative of islet graft function, was shown to last longer in the more recent period, too [10].

The overall clinical condition of islet recipients improved after transplantation. After the transplant, islet recipients record less episodes of hypoglycemia [11], and they become more sensitive to and aware of hypoglycemia. There are also numerous reports of onset reduction and/or slowing progression of chronic complications of diabetes [12]. Islet transplantation stabilizes hemostatic abnormalities and cerebral metabolism, improves diastolic function and QT dispersion, delays arterial intima and media thickening, reduces the progression of diabetic retinopathy and improves nerve conduction velocity. In islet and kidney recipients, it prolongs graft survival and prevents the reduction in vascular function of the kidney graft. In a small number of transplanted patients, a low number of cardiovascular deaths was observed during a 10-year follow-up, too [12].

Most of the effects were evidenced not only in patients with complete insulin independency, but also in those with partial transplant function. The effects so far observed could be secondary to such an improved metabolic control as demonstrated by the significant reduction in blood glucose levels and HbA1c as well as to the presence of circulating C-peptide [12]. Many data suggested that C-peptide may have a direct effect on the tissues subjected to chronic complications. The consequence of islet transplantation positive effects is a better quality of life both in insulin-free patients and in patients with partial graft function [13]. Taken together, these results lead to pose that the aim of the transplant is not so much the complete insulin independence, but the gain of better metabolic control and the reduction in acute complications.

While islet transplantation significantly improves glycemic control and the quality of life of the patient and positively affects diabetic complications, the problems associated with transplantation should be considered, too. The complications of a transplant procedure are mainly the risk of portal thrombosis caused by the islet injection in the hepatic flow and bleeding caused by entering the catheter through the liver [10]. Bleeding risk has much improved today by closing the entry site of the catheter [14]. Intravascular thrombosis is infrequent, unless more than 10 ml of tissue be injected. The islets produce factors that trigger intravascular coagulation and an inflammatory process [15]. If severe thrombosis is rare, microthromboses are more frequent and occur at the level of hepatic sinusoids and terminal portal branches, leading to increased portal pressure after the transplant. This phenomenon limits the number of infusions to 3–4 which can be repeated in the same patient, those who do not gain complete insulin independence through one single islet infusion or who undergo graft exhaustion during follow-up.

Immunosuppressive therapy, in order to avoid rejection and recurrence of autoimmunity, is the real problem of isolated islet transplantation. Effective immunosuppressive therapies are similar to those required for the organ transplant in toto [16]. It is well known that immunosuppression is burdened by severe side effects (mainly infections, nephrotoxicity, leukopenia and neoplasia). The essential components of immunosuppressive therapy are calcineurin inhibitors (usually tacrolimus) and mycophenolate. Induction with antilymphocyte serum or anti-IL-2 monoclonal antibody is also common practice. In recent years, several reports highlighted the need for anti-inflammatory strategies to reduce inflammation induced by islets themselves that hinders islet engraftment. Among the efficient strategies, there are anti-TNF drugs or reparixin [16, 17]. Islet engraftment improvement was even reported thanks to the peritransplant use of GLP-1 analogues that reduce the metabolic demand and stress of the newly transplanted β cells [18].

## Current Clinical Indications of Islet Transplantation in Pediatric Practice

Islet transplantation has already been successfully performed in children. So far, only islet autotransplantation has been performed in children and young people suffering from chronic pancreatitis. These are a limited number of cases. Two recent case reports published from major centers with an active program of pediatric autotransplantation describe dozens of treated patients. In particular, the University of Minnesota reported islet autotransplantation in 75 pediatric patients [19] and the University of Cincinnati in 14 [20]. Their average age is around 13–15 years. The causes that led to the transplant are mostly idiopathic, cystic fibrosis or other genetic forms. The isolation procedure is very complex due to the fibrotic conditions of digested pancreas and the fragility of the pancreatic islets in young patients; due to the small size of the organs, the number of isolated islets is often very low. Over the last few years, several changes to traditional isolation procedures have been proposed for the pancreas of children and young people suffering from chronic pancreatitis thus improving the isolation outcomes [21].

The primary goal of surgical treatment of chronic pancreatitis in childhood is pain relieve and restoration of quality of life. After pancreatectomy, chronic pain was alleviated in the majority of patients, as documented by the high percentage of narcotic-independent patients. An improved postoperative quality of life was also reported, with a return to daily activities as the participation in extracurricular activities, attending school, and progressing social and physical development [19, 20].

The addition of islet autotransplantation to total pancreatectomy did not increase the morbidity associated with total pancreatectomy alone. Indeed, islet autotransplantation can achieve acceptable long-term glycemic control. The insulin independence rate is about 41% according to the University of Minnesota and about 29% according to the University of Cincinnati experience. Younger children (<12 years) were more likely to achieve insulin independence than older children (overall insulin independence rate in 5- to 12-year-old patients is >50%). In this experience, insulin independence has been observed for as long as 10 years. Of the 31 patients who attained insulin independence, only 3 reverted to insulin dependence during follow-up. Most patients achieved stable glycemic control and there was no incidence of 'brittle' diabetes or severe hypoglycemic events requiring urgent medical evaluation.

Injection of isolated islets into the muscle is proposed when intraportal autotransplantation is not feasible. Total pancreatectomy and later islet transplantation was performed in a 7-year-old girl with hereditary pancreatitis with the common trypsin mutation, R122H, suffering from repeated abdominal pains, severe acute pancreatitis and septic episodes [22]. The choice of the intramuscular site and not the intrahepatic one is due to the fact that the exocrine part of the pancreatic tissue might create an abnormal microenvironment if transplanted into the liver. A total of 163,000 islet equivalents (6,400 islet/kg body weight) were transplanted within the fibers of the brachioradialis muscle of the right forearm. After the transplant, her quality of life greatly improved and she gained 8 kg in weight. An adequate islet function was observed; 2 years later she had an optimal HbA1c (5.3%) with insulin requirements of 0.18 units/kg/day, compared to 0.75 immediately after operation with preserved C-peptide levels.

Islet autotransplantation after total pancreatectomy in pediatric patients appeared therefore to be a feasible therapeutic option. In painful chronic pancreatitis leading to a decreasing quality of life and affecting emotional, social and physical development of the child, the surgical approach appears to be the best option. In the presence of a large pancreatic duct, a resection/decompression procedure should be preferred. In case of a small duct that makes a decompression procedure quite ineffective, total pancreatectomy and islet autotransplantation is recommended.

## Perspectives in Islet Transplantation

Today, islet transplantation may greatly improve glucose control for many years in patients affected by insulin-dependent diabetes mellitus (type 1 or secondary); immunosuppression therapy is required outside autotransplantation. Matters of research are improvements in islet engraftment in order to prolong graft function, reduction or even abrogation of immunosuppression therapy, and extension of this procedure to a great population, both adult and pediatric.

The control of the alloreaction toward the graft and the autoimmunity is a key point for the success and safety of islet transplantation. The use of highly potent and selective drugs for the initiation and maintenance of immunosuppression has made significant progress in reducing the frequency of acute rejection, thus prolonging graft survival [2]. The early depletion of alloreactive T cells appears to be a key point. This promotes a hyporesponsive environment and peripheral mechanisms of anergy, which are requirements for the onset of tolerance. A high rate of long-term insulin independence has been made possible through agents that induce T-cell depletion such as alemtuzumab. Co-stimulation blockage using belatacept together with T-cell depletion increases the rate of insulin independence with islets from a single donor and prolongs allograft survival, too. It is well known that the current immunosuppression therapies are hampered by severe side effects both in brief and long-term follow-ups. The real challenge is to offer the patients a safe therapy by reducing immunosuppressant toxicity. A tolerogenic regimen that might utilize more selective biologics and techniques that might target only donor-specific reactive T cells while expanding populations of regulatory T cells should determine a real progress in the pharmacological treatment of islet allotransplantation [23].

To improve Islet engraftment and in vivo function, a large number of islets has to be infused: in fact, with current isolation and implantation procedures, almost half of the islets is lost within a few hours after infusion due to an aspecific inflammatory reaction around the islets. Islets are usually transplanted into the portal vein by percutaneous transhepatic injection. This is a minimally invasive procedure that allows the islets to be immediately perfused by the portal flow spreading into a large space as the hepatic vessel network is. However, following infusion into the portal vessels, islets are involved in a nonspecific inflammatory and thrombotic reaction that destroys islets [15]. Subsequently, in the portal circulation, islets are chronically exposed to high drug concentrations and high levels of nutrients and gut hormones resulting in insulin hypersecretion. Alternative sites for islet transplantation have been, therefore, proposed [24]. Numerous sites have been proposed and tested, both experimentally and in some cases clinically, including spleen, kidney subcapsule, muscles, bone marrow, omentum, gastrointestinal wall and subcutaneous spaces [25]. The bone marrow was proposed as an interesting option: it is a protected and extravascular but also well-perfused site, which is suitable for co-transplantation of islets with immunomodulatory cells, such as T-regulatory cells or mesenchymal stem cells, which could help to prevent auto- and alloimmune responses [25]. Alternative approaches have been the pre-implantation and vascularization of subcutaneous devices or encapsulation of islets [24]. Also, intramuscular or subcutaneous islet implantation was shown to allow co-implantation of cells and devices for favoring islet engraftment, immunomodulation or immunoprotection.

Independent clinical trials are now testing the real clinical feasibility of these two approaches.

The real feasibility of islet transplantation in a large number of patients depends on the availability of a large number of β cells. With the purpose of offering a therapeutic strategy to many patients, alternative sources of insulin-producing cells are now under study. Many attempts have been made up to now, the main ones using human embryonic stem cells or pancreatic duct cells [26]. Alternatively, the transdifferentiation of acinar or hepatic cells to β cells has been proposed [27].

## Conclusions

Islet transplantation now offers a possible solution for selected patients affected by brittle type 1 diabetes mellitus or by secondary diabetes mellitus after total pancreatectomy. Many attempts are now being carried out in order to find solutions to the current problems facing islet transplantation, from the toxicity of the immunosuppressive therapy to the limited graft function and duration. The hope is that these procedures will allow a safe and feasible therapeutic option for an increasing number of patients suffering from diabetes mellitus without any age range restrictions.

## References


1 Niclauss N, Morel P, Berney T: Has the gap between pancreas and islet transplantation closed? Transplantation 2014;98:593–599.

2 Bruni A, Gala-Lopez B, Pepper AR, Abualhassan NS, Shapiro AJ: Islet cell transplantation for the treatment of type 1 diabetes: recent advances and future challenges. Diabetes Metab Syndr Obes 2014;7:211–223.

3 Radomski M, Zureikat AH: Total pancreatectomy and islet cell autotransplantation: outcomes, controversies and new techniques. JOP 2015;31:1–10.

4 Dong M, Parsaik AK, Erwin PJ, Farnell MB, Murad MH, Kudva YC: Systematic review and meta-analysis: islet autotransplantation after pancreatectomy for minimizing diabetes. Clin Endocrinol (Oxf) 2011;75:771–779.

5 Naziruddin B, Matsumoto S, Noguchi H, Takita M, Shimoda M, Fujita Y, Chujo D, Tate C, Onaca N, Lamont J, Kobayashi N, Levy MF: Improved pancreatic islet isolation outcome in autologous transplantation for chronic pancreatitis. Cell Transplant 2012; 21:553–558.

6 Lysy PA, Weir GC, Bonner-Weir S: Concise review: pancreas regeneration: recent advances and perspectives. Stem Cells Transl Med 2012;1:150–159.

7 Wilson GC, Sutton JM, Abbott DE, Smith MT, Lowy AM, Matthews JB, Rilo HL, Schmulewitz N, Salehi M, Choe K, Brunner J, Hanseman DJ, Sussman JJ, Edwards MJ, Ahmad SA: Long-term outcomes after total pancreatectomy and islet cell autotransplantation: is it a durable operation? Ann Surg 2014;260:659–665.

8 Balzano G, Piemonti L: Autologous islet transplantation in patients requiring pancreatectomy for neoplasm. Curr Diab Rep 2014;14:512.

9 Bertuzzi F, Verzaro R, Provenzano V, Ricordi C: Brittle type 1 diabetes mellitus. Curr Med Chem 2007;14:1739–1744.

10 Balamurugan AN, Naziruddin B, Lockridge A, Tiwari M, Loganathan G, Takita M, Matsumoto S, Papas K, Trieger M, Rainis H, Kin T, Kay TW, Wease S, Messinger S, Ricordi C, Alejandro R, Markmann J, Kerr-Conti J, Rickels MR, Liu C, Zhang X, Witkowski P, Posselt A, Maffi P, Secchi A, Berney T, O'Connell PJ, Hering BJ, Barton FB: Islet product characteristics and factors related to successful human islet transplantation from the Collaborative Islet Transplant Registry (CITR) 1999–2010. Am J Transplant 2014;14:2595–2606.

11 Vantyghem MC, Raverdy V, Balavoine AS, Defrance F, Caiazzo R, Arnalsteen L, Gmyr V, Hazzan M, Noël C, Kerr-Conte J, Pattou F: Continuous glucose monitoring after islet transplantation in type 1 diabetes: an excellent graft function (β-score greater than 7) is required to abrogate hyperglycemia, whereas a minimal function is necessary to suppress severe hypoglycemia (β-score greater than 3). J Clin Endocrinol Metab 2012;97:E2078–E2083.
12 Fiorina P, Shapiro AM, Ricordi C, Secchi A: The clinical impact of islet transplantation. Am J Transplant 2008;8:1990–1997.
13 Tharavanij T, Betancourt A, Messinger S, Cure P, Leitao CB, Baidal DA, Froud T, Ricordi C, Alejandro R: Improved long-term health-related quality of life after islet transplantation. Transplantation 2008;86:1161–1167.
14 Froud T, Yrizarry JM, Alejandro R, Ricordi C: Use of D-STAT to prevent bleeding following percutaneous transhepatic intraportal islet transplantation. Cell Transplant 2004;13:55–59.
15 Johansson H, Lukinius A, Moberg L, Lundgren T, Berne C, Foss A, Felldin M, Källen R, Salmela K, Tibell A, Tufveson G, Ekdahl KN, Elgue G, Korsgren O, Nilsson B: Tissue factor produced by the endocrine cells of the islets of Langerhans is associated with a negative outcome of clinical islet transplantation. Diabetes 2005;54:1755–1762.
16 Bellin MD, Barton FB, Heitman A, Harmon JV, Kandaswamy R, Balamurugan AN, Sutherland DE, Alejandro R, Hering BJ: Potent induction immunotherapy promotes long-term insulin independence after islet transplantation in type 1 diabetes. Am J Transplant 2012;12:1576–1583.
17 Citro A, Cantarelli E, Maffi P, Nano R, Melzi R, Mercalli A, Dugnani E, Sordi V, Magistretti P, Daffonchio L, Ruffini PA, Allegretti M, Secchi A, Bonifacio E, Piemonti L: CXCR1/2 inhibition enhances pancreatic islet survival after transplantation. J Clin Invest 2012;122:3647–3651.
18 Wang Y, Qi M, McGarrigle JJ, Rady B, Davis ME, Vaca P, Oberholzer J: Use of glucagon-like peptide-1 agonists to improve islet graft performance. Curr Diab Rep 2013;13:723–732.
19 Chinnakotla S, Bellin MD, Schwarzenberg SJ, Radosevich DM, Cook M, Dunn TB, Beilman GJ, Freeman ML, Balamurugan AN, Wilhelm J, Bland B, Jimenez-Vega JM, Hering BJ, Vickers SM, Pruett TL, Sutherland DE: Total pancreatectomy and islet autotransplantation in children for chronic pancreatitis: indication, surgical techniques, postoperative management, and long-term outcomes. Ann Surg 2014;260:56–64.
20 Wilson GC, Sutton JM, Salehi M, Schmulewitz N, Smith MT, Kucera S, Choe KA, Brunner JE, Abbott DE, Sussman JJ, Ahmad SA: Surgical outcomes after total pancreatectomy and islet cell autotransplantation in pediatric patients. Surgery 2013;154:777–783.
21 Bottino R, Bertera S, Grupillo M, Melvin PR, Humar A, Mazariegos G, Moser AJ, Walsh RM, Fung J, Gelrud A, Slivka A, Soltys K, Wijkstrom M, Trucco M: Isolation of human islets for autologous islet transplantation in children and adolescents with chronic pancreatitis. J Transplant 2012;2012:642787.
22 Rafael E, Tibell A, Rydén M, Lundgren T, Sävendahl L, Borgström B, Arnelo U, Isaksson B, Nilsson B, Korsgren O, Permert J: Intramuscular autotransplantation of pancreatic islets in a 7-year-old child: a 2-year follow-up. Am J Transplant 2008;8:458–862.
23 Ricordi C: The path for tolerance permissive immunomodulation in islet transplantation. Transplantation 2014;98:1260–1261.
24 Smink AM, Faas MM, de Vos P: Toward engineering a novel transplantation site for human pancreatic islets. Diabetes 2013;62:1357–1364.
25 Cantarelli E, Piemonti L: Alternative transplantation sites for pancreatic islet grafts. Curr Diab Rep 2011;11:364–374.
26 Ricordi C, Inverardi L, Domínguez-Bendala J: From cellular therapies to tissue reprogramming and regenerative strategies in the treatment of diabetes. Regen Med 2012;7(6 suppl):41–48.
27 Lysy PA, Weir GC, Bonner-Weir S: Making β cells from adult cells within the pancreas. Curr Diab Rep 2013;13:695–703.

Federico Bertuzzi, MD
Diabetology Unit, Niguarda Hospital
Piazza Ospedale Maggiore 3, IT–20162 Milan (Italy)
E-Mail federico.bertuzzi@ospedaleniguarda.it

Cappa M, Cianfarani S, Ghizzoni L, Loche S, Maghnie M (eds): Advanced Therapies in Pediatric Endocrinology and Diabetology. Endocr Dev. Basel, Karger, 2016, vol 30, pp 23–28 (DOI: 10.1159/000439323)

# Glucagon-Like Peptide-1 Receptor Agonist Treatment for Pediatric Obesity

Aaron S. Kelly

Departments of Pediatrics and Medicine, University of Minnesota Medical School, and University of Minnesota Masonic Children's Hospital, Minneapolis, Minn., USA

**Abstract**

Obesity is a complex and retractable disease for which effective and durable treatments are elusive. Successful treatment of severe obesity with lifestyle modification therapy alone is highly unlikely, particularly for adolescents. Pharmacotherapy, if appropriately prescribed, can be an effective tool to use in conjunction with lifestyle modification therapy to achieve better weight loss outcomes. Only a few obesity medications have been evaluated in children and adolescents with results suggesting modest efficacy. However, a new pipeline of obesity drugs has been recently approved for use among adults. Among these, glucagon-like peptide-1 receptor agonist (GLP-1RA) treatment appears to have reasonable weight loss efficacy along with other beneficial pleiotropic effects. Although larger trials will be required to confirm the results, two small pediatric clinical trials have suggested that GLP-1RA treatment may be useful in adolescents with severe obesity. Once sufficient evidence is generated supporting the safety and efficacy of GLP-1RAs and other obesity medications in youth, the pediatric medical community needs to become less resistant to the use of pharmacotherapy. Otherwise, poor outcomes will continue to be the norm. 

Effective and durable treatments for pediatric obesity remain elusive. This is particularly true for youth with severe obesity, defined as a body mass index (BMI) ≥120% of the 95th percentile or BMI ≥35 [1]. Severe obesity is the fastest growing category of pediatric obesity and the prevalence in the United States is estimated to be approximately 6% among youth 2–19 years old [2]. Children and adolescents with severe obesity are highly likely to carry their excess adiposity into adulthood [3]. Therefore, instituting appropriately intensive treatments in childhood is imperative. Although lifestyle modification therapy (dietary, physical activity and behavioral counseling) appears to be somewhat effective if implemented in younger children with severe obesity [4], its effect in adolescents is minimal [5]. In fact, only 2% of adolescents with severe obesity are able to lose and maintain a clinically meaningful amount of weight with lifestyle modification therapy alone [5]. By far the most effective treatment for severe obesity in adolescents is bariatric surgery [6, 7]. However, access is limited (primarily by lack of insurance coverage), risks of surgery are greater than that of lifestyle modification or pharmacotherapy, and most adolescents (and their families) are unwilling to submit to this invasive treatment option.

Bridging the wide weight loss effectiveness gap separating lifestyle modification therapy and bariatric surgery should be a major medical priority in the field of pediatrics, and pharmacotherapy is a highly promising treatment approach for narrowing that gap. However, only one medication, orlistat, is currently approved by the United States Food and Drug Administration for the treatment of obesity in adolescents 12 years of age and older. Orlistat, however, is far from an ideal agent because of its relatively modest efficacy (BMI reduction of approximately 3%) and often intolerable side effects such as fecal urgency, oily spotting and fatty stools [8]. Although not approved to treat obesity, metformin is another medication that has been evaluated for its weight loss effects among children and adolescents. The efficacy of metformin is similar to orlistat (approximately 3% BMI reduction) and studies have reported minimal to no improvements in cardiometabolic risk factors [9, 10]. It should be noted, though, that since adult trials have demonstrated a reduction in the risk of type 2 diabetes development, metformin may have some value beyond BMI reduction for youth with obesity at high risk of developing the disease [11].

Despite the lack of available medication for the treatment of pediatric obesity, the adult pharmaceutical pipeline offers hope that new agents will soon be available for pediatric use. Indeed, over the last few years, the United States Food and Drug Administration has approved four new obesity medications for use in adults: lorcaserin, the combination of phentermine and topiramate, the combination of naltrexone and bupropion, and high-dose liraglutide. The placebo-subtracted reduction in body weight for these drugs range from 3 to 9% depending upon the specific medication and dose used [12]. It is hoped that all of these agents will be evaluated in pediatric trials in the near future.

Of these new medications, one of the most effective in terms of weight loss and cardiometabolic risk factor improvement is the glucagon-like peptide-1 receptor agonist (GLP-1RA) class. GLP-1RAs were originally developed for the treatment of type 2 diabetes. However, in addition to improving glycemic control, GLP-1RAs reduce body weight, which has subsequently been demonstrated in a number of adult trials [13]. Two independent trials among adults with obesity but without type 2 diabetes demonstrated that exenatide reduced body weight by approximately 3% over treatment periods ranging from 4 to 6 months [14, 15]. In two separate reports of the same phase II trial [16, 17], high-dose liraglutide was shown to significantly reduce body weight for up to 2 years among adults with obesity. Evidence suggests that GLP-1RAs reduce appetite by acting on receptors in the hypothalamus, and also enhance satiety signaling via peripheral (slowing of gastric emptying) and central (augmentation of distention signals from the gut to the nucleus tractus solitarius region of the hindbrain) pathways [18–20]. Perhaps GLP-1RAs also increase resting energy expenditure [21]; however, this has not been a consistent finding [22, 23]. In addition, there is some evidence that GLP-1RAs blunt the reduction in leptin that often occurs in parallel with weight loss, which might bode well in terms of weight loss maintenance [24].

To date, only two studies have evaluated the weight loss effects of GLP-1RAs among youth. The first was a randomized, controlled, crossover trial in 12 adolescents who received either exenatide or the control condition (lifestyle modification therapy) for 3 months, and were then crossed over to the other condition [25]. BMI was significantly reduced by approximately 5% in the exenatide phase versus control phase. In addition to weight loss, improvements were observed in glucose tolerance and surrogate measures of insulin sensitivity and β-cell function. The second trial utilized a double-blind, randomized, placebo-controlled design and assigned 26 adolescents with severe obesity to either exenatide or matching placebo for 3 months, followed by an open label extension during which all patients received exenatide treatment [26]. The placebo-subtracted BMI reduction with exenatide in this trial was approximately 3% at the 3-month time point. Among patients who received exenatide treatment for the entire 6 months of the trial, BMI was reduced by approximately 4%. In addition, a clinically meaningful reduction in systolic blood pressure (approximately 6 mm Hg) was observed. Although short-term results with GLP-1RAs appear favorable, follow-up trials will need to evaluate whether BMI reduction continues beyond 3 months and assess whether weight loss is sustained over time. Future pediatric trials should also seek to characterize the pleiotropic effects, beyond weight reduction, that accompany GLP-1RA treatment. These include potential improvements in glucose tolerance, insulin resistance, blood pressure, vascular dysfunction and inflammation [25, 27–30].

Nausea, which is often mild and transient in most individuals, is the most common adverse effect of GLP-1RAs. Evidence is mixed regarding whether acute pancreatitis is associated with GLP-1RA treatment, and most of the data come from studies involving adults with type 2 diabetes, a disease known to increase the risk of pancreatitis. Many studies have reported no association between GLP-1RA use and pancreatitis [31–34]; however, others have suggested a link [35, 36]. Results from ongoing GLP-1RA cardiovascular outcome trials, which are prospectively tracking pancreatitis incidence, are eagerly anticipated as data should clarify this important safety issue.

The field of pediatric obesity medicine is entering an exciting period as a burgeoning pipeline of obesity medications is beginning to emerge. It is hoped that clinical trials assessing pharmacotherapies for pediatric obesity will soon be initiated, including studies evaluating the safety and efficacy of GLP-1RAs. For many youth, especially those afflicted with severe obesity, combination pharmacotherapy (targeting multiple mechanisms) will likely be the most effective medical approach. Studies addressing tailored medicine will be important, and these trials should focus on identifying factors associated with response and nonresponse to treatment. The right combination of obesity medications used in the right pediatric patients could go a long way in bridging the large efficacy gap separating lifestyle modification from bariatric surgery. However, pharmacotherapy should be viewed as a tool to be used in conjunction with intensive lifestyle modification, as the latter should always serve as the foundation of proper obesity management.

## Disclosure Statement

Dr. Kelly serves on a pediatric obesity advisory committee for Takeda Pharmaceuticals and for Novo Nordisk Pharmaceuticals but does not receive personal or professional income for his services. Dr. Kelly received research support (in the form of drug and placebo) from Amylin Pharmaceuticals for some of the work reported in this article.

## References

1 Kelly AS, Barlow SE, Rao G, Inge TH, Hayman LL, Steinberger J, Urbina EM, Ewing LJ, Daniels SR: Severe obesity in children and adolescents: identification, associated health risks, and treatment approaches: a scientific statement from the American Heart Association. Circulation 2013;128:1689–1712.

2 Skinner AC, Skelton JA: Prevalence and trends in obesity and severe obesity among children in the United States, 1999–2012. JAMA Pediatr 2014;168: 561–566.

3 Freedman DS, Mei Z, Srinivasan SR, Berenson GS, Dietz WH: Cardiovascular risk factors and excess adiposity among overweight children and adolescents: the Bogalusa Heart Study. J Pediatr 2007;150: 12–17.

4 Knop C, Singer V, Uysal Y, Schaefer A, Wolters B, Reinehr T: Extremely obese children respond better than extremely obese adolescents to lifestyle interventions. Pediatr Obes 2015;10:7–14.

5 Danielsson P, Kowalski J, Ekblom O, Marcus C: Response of severely obese children and adolescents to behavioral treatment. Arch Pediatr Adolesc Med 2012;166:1103–1108.

6 Alqahtani AR, Antonisamy B, Alamri H, Elahmedi M, Zimmerman VA: Laparoscopic sleeve gastrectomy in 108 obese children and adolescents aged 5 to 21 years. Ann Surg 2012;256:266–273.

7 Inge TH, Jenkins TM, Zeller M, Dolan L, Daniels SR, Garcia VF, Brandt ML, Bean J, Gamm K, Xanthakos SA: Baseline BMI is a strong predictor of nadir BMI after adolescent gastric bypass. J Pediatr 2010;156: 103–108.

8 Chanoine JP, Hampl S, Jensen C, Boldrin M, Hauptman J: Effect of orlistat on weight and body composition in obese adolescents: a randomized controlled trial. JAMA 2005;293:2873–2883.

9 Wilson DM, Abrams SH, Aye T, Lee PD, Lenders C, Lustig RH, Osganian SV, Feldman HA; Glaser Pediatric Research Network Obesity Study Group: Metformin extended release treatment of adolescent obesity: a 48-week randomized, double-blind, placebo-controlled trial with 48-week follow-up. Arch Pediatr Adolesc Med 2010;164:116–123.

10 Yanovski JA, Krakoff J, Salaita CG, McDuffie JR, Kozlosky M, Sebring NG, Reynolds JC, Brady SM, Calis KA: Effects of metformin on body weight and body composition in obese insulin-resistant children: a randomized clinical trial. Diabetes 2011;60: 477–485.

11 Knowler WC, Barrett-Connor E, Fowler SE, Hamman RF, Lachin JM, Walker EA, Nathan DM: Reduction in the incidence of type 2 diabetes with lifestyle intervention or metformin. N Engl J Med 2002; 346:393–403.
12 Yanovski SZ, Yanovski JA: Long-term drug treatment for obesity: a systematic and clinical review. JAMA 2014;311:74–86.
13 Vilsboll T, Christensen M, Junker AE, Knop FK, Gluud LL: Effects of glucagon-like peptide-1 receptor agonists on weight loss: systematic review and meta-analyses of randomised controlled trials. BMJ 2012;344:d7771.
14 Rosenstock J, Klaff LJ, Schwartz S, Northrup J, Holcombe JH, Wilhelm K, Trautmann M: Effects of exenatide and lifestyle modification on body weight and glucose tolerance in obese subjects with and without pre-diabetes. Diabetes Care 2010;33:1173–1175.
15 Dushay J, Gao C, Gopalakrishnan GS, Crawley M, Mitten EK, Wilker E, Mullington J, Maratos-Flier E: Short-term exenatide treatment leads to significant weight loss in a subset of obese women without diabetes. Diabetes Care 2012;35:4–11.
16 Astrup A, Rössner S, Van Gaal L, Rissanen A, Niskanen L, Al Hakim M, Madsen J, Rasmussen MF, Lean ME: Effects of liraglutide in the treatment of obesity: a randomised, double-blind, placebo-controlled study. Lancet 2009;374:1606–1616.
17 Astrup A, Carraro R, Finer N, Harper A, Kunesova M, Lean ME, Niskanen L, Rasmussen MF, Rissanen A, Rössner S, Savolainen MJ, Van Gaal L: Safety, tolerability and sustained weight loss over 2 years with the once-daily human GLP-1 analogue, liraglutide. Int J Obes (Lond) 2012;36:843–854.
18 Bojanowska E: Physiology and pathophysiology of glucagon-like peptide-1 (GLP-1): the role of GLP-1 in the pathogenesis of diabetes mellitus, obesity, and stress. Med Sci Monit 2005;11:RA271–RA278.
19 Edwards CM, Stanley SA, Davis R, Brynes AE, Frost GS, Seal LJ, Ghatei MA, Bloom SR: Exendin-4 reduces fasting and postprandial glucose and decreases energy intake in healthy volunteers. Am J Physiol Endocrinol Metab 2001;281:E155–E161.
20 Grill HJ, Hayes MR: The nucleus tractus solitarius: a portal for visceral afferent signal processing, energy status assessment and integration of their combined effects on food intake. Int J Obes (Lond) 2009; 33(suppl 1):S11–S15.
21 Horowitz M, Flint A, Jones KL, Hindsberger C, Rasmussen MF, Kapitza C, Doran S, Jax T, Zdravkovic M, Chapman IM: Effect of the once-daily human GLP-1 analogue liraglutide on appetite, energy intake, energy expenditure and gastric emptying in type 2 diabetes. Diabetes Res Clin Pract 2012;97: 258–266.
22 Bradley DP, Kulstad R, Racine N, Shenker Y, Meredith M, Schoeller DA: Alterations in energy balance following exenatide administration. Appl Physiol Nutr Metab 2012;37:893–899.
23 Harder H, Nielsen L, Tu DT, Astrup A: The effect of liraglutide, a long-acting glucagon-like peptide 1 derivative, on glycemic control, body composition, and 24-h energy expenditure in patients with type 2 diabetes. Diabetes Care 2004;27:1915–1921.
24 Iepsen EW, Lundgren J, Dirksen C, Jensen JE, Pedersen O, Hansen T, Madsbad S, Holst JJ, Torekov SS: Treatment with a GLP-1 receptor agonist diminishes the decrease in free plasma leptin during maintenance of weight loss. Int J Obes (Lond) 2015;39:834–841.
25 Kelly AS, Metzig AM, Rudser KD, Fitch AK, Fox CK, Nathan BM, Deering M, Schwartz BL, Abuzzahab MJ, Gandrud LM, Moran A, Billington CJ, Schwarzenberg SJ: Exenatide as a weight-loss therapy in extreme pediatric obesity: a randomized, controlled pilot study. Obesity (Silver Spring) 2012;20: 364–370.
26 Kelly AS, Rudser KD, Nathan BM, Fox CK, Metzig AM, Coombes BJ, Fitch AK, Bomberg EM, Abuzzahab MJ: The effect of glucagon-like peptide-1 receptor agonist therapy on body mass index in adolescents with severe obesity: a randomized, placebo-controlled, clinical trial. JAMA Pediatr 2013;167:355–360.
27 Chaudhuri A, Ghanim H, Vora M, Sia CL, Korzeniewski K, Dhindsa S, Makdissi A, Dandona P: Exenatide exerts a potent antiinflammatory effect. J Clin Endocrinol Metab 2012;97:198–207.
28 Koska J, Schwartz EA, Mullin MP, Schwenke DC, Reaven PD: Improvement of postprandial endothelial function after a single dose of exenatide in individuals with impaired glucose tolerance and recent-onset type 2 diabetes. Diabetes Care 2010;33: 1028–1030.
29 Okerson T, Yan P, Stonehouse A, Brodows R: Effects of exenatide on systolic blood pressure in subjects with type 2 diabetes. Am J Hypertens 2010;23:334–339.
30 Yamazaki S, Satoh H, Watanabe T: Liraglutide enhances insulin sensitivity by activating AMP-activated protein kinase in male Wistar rats. Endocrinology 2014;155:3288–3301.
31 Alves C, Batel-Marques F, Macedo AF: A meta-analysis of serious adverse events reported with exenatide and liraglutide: acute pancreatitis and cancer. Diabetes Res Clin Pract 2012;98:271–284.
32 Garg R, Chen W, Pendergrass M: Acute pancreatitis in type 2 diabetes treated with exenatide or sitagliptin: a retrospective observational pharmacy claims analysis. Diabetes Care 2010;33:2349–2354.

33 Romley JA, Goldman DP, Solomon M, McFadden D, Peters AL: Exenatide therapy and the risk of pancreatitis and pancreatic cancer in a privately insured population. Diabetes Technol Ther 2012;14:904–911.
34 Wenten M, Gaebler JA, Hussein M, Pelletier EM, Smith DB, Girase P, Noel RA, Braun DK, Bloomgren GL: Relative risk of acute pancreatitis in initiators of exenatide twice daily compared with other anti-diabetic medication: a follow-up study. Diabet Med 2012;29:1412–1418.
35 Elashoff M, Matveyenko AV, Gier B, Elashoff R, Butler PC: Pancreatitis, pancreatic, and thyroid cancer with glucagon-like peptide-1-based therapies. Gastroenterology 2011;141:150–156.
36 Singh S, Chang HY, Richards TM, Weiner JP, Clark JM, Segal JB: Glucagonlike peptide 1-based therapies and risk of hospitalization for acute pancreatitis in type 2 diabetes mellitus: a population-based matched case-control study. JAMA Intern Med 2013;173:534–539.

Aaron S. Kelly, PhD
Department of Pediatrics, University of Minnesota Medical School
420 Delaware Street SE, MMC 715
Minneapolis, MN 55455 (USA)
E-Mail kelly105@umn.edu

Cappa M, Cianfarani S, Ghizzoni L, Loche S, Maghnie M (eds): Advanced Therapies in Pediatric Endocrinology and Diabetology. Endocr Dev. Basel, Karger, 2016, vol 30, pp 29–36 (DOI: 10.1159/000439324)

# Docosahexaenoic Acid and Its Role in G-Protein-Coupled Receptor 120 Activation in Children Affected by Nonalcoholic Fatty Liver Disease

Claudia Della Corte[a] · Antonella Mosca[a] · Aurelio Ionata[b] · Valerio Nobili[a]

[a]Hepato-Metabolic Disease Unit, Bambino Gesù Children's Hospital, IRCCS, Rome, and [b]Azienda Sanitaria Regionale del Molise (A.S.Re.M), Isernia, Italy

**Abstract**

Nonalcoholic fatty liver disease (NAFLD) is one of the most important causes of chronic liver disease in children and adults. Recently, therapeutic supplementation with docosahexaenoic acid (DHA) showed an anti-inflammatory and insulin-sensitizing effect in children with NAFLD. The anti-inflammatory effects of DHA depend on its ability to alter phospholipid composition of the cell membrane, to disrupt lipid rafts and to hamper the transcriptional activity of nuclear factor-κB that controls the expression of proinflammatory cytokines. These effects of DHA are due to the interaction with the G-protein-coupled receptor 120 (GRP120), a lipid-sensing receptor highly expressed in activated macrophages. In fact, DHA may activate GPR120 expression in macrophages causing anti-inflammatory effects, and insulin-sensitizing and antidiabetic effects in vivo. Recently, it has been shown that GPR120 is also expressed by the Kupffer cells of the liver. A diet low in n-3 polyunsaturated fatty acids, as well as the presence of genetic factors, may induce a reduction in the GRP120 signal and the activation of Kupffer cells and inflammation during NAFLD. Therefore, it is conceivable that DHA/GRP120 may play a key role in slowing the progression of liver damage in patients with NAFLD.



During the last decade, ω-3 (n-3) polyunsaturated fatty acids (PUFAs) have received particular attention for their abilities to counteract inflammation, oxidative stress, angiogenesis and metastasis [1]. The balance between n-3 and n-6 PUFAs is crucial to maintain metabolic homeostasis and a high n-6/n-3 ratio, as that caused by Western diets, may promote the pathogenesis of many diseases [2]. These properties provide a scientific rationale to explain the beneficial effects of n-3 PUFAs in several chronic diseases, including diabetes mellitus type 2, cardiovascular diseases and cancers [3–5]. The most studied n-3 PUFAs in clinical applications, eicosapentaenoic acid, docosapentaenoic acid and docosahexaenoic acid (DHA), are primarily contained in fish oil, but marine algae and phytoplankton are also relevant sources of n-3 PUFAs. Furthermore, it has been reported that n-3 PUFAs, particularly DHA, may exert their anti-inflammatory and insulin-sensitizing effects by interacting with G-protein-coupled receptor 120 (GPR120), a lipid-sensing receptor highly expressed in activated macrophages [6].

Interestingly, recently, the therapeutic value of n-3 PUFA supplementation has been investigated in adult subjects affected by nonalcoholic fatty liver disease (NAFLD) [7]. NAFLD is a multifactorial condition including a wide spectrum of liver damage which includes simple steatosis, steatohepatitis and eventually fibrosis [8]. Current epidemiological evidence has highlighted that NAFLD has to be considered the most common cause of chronic liver disease in children and adults, which is becoming a major public health problem economically afflicting westernized countries [9, 10].

The purpose of the present minireview is to provide an overview on the role of DHA in liver metabolism and the clinical significance of this natural agent in the treatment of pediatric NAFLD.

## Mechanism of Docosahexaenoic Acid and G-Protein-Coupled Receptor 120

DHA, which is the longest-chain and most unsaturated fatty acid commonly found in biological systems, is detected at high levels only in specific tissues of mammals, such as the retinal rod outer segment and synaptosomes. However, in other tissues, DHA can be enriched through dietary supplementation with food that contains a large quantity of this n-3 PUFA, such as fish oil and marine algae [11]. In mammals, DHA exerts its action mainly on the cell membrane where it is known to be readily incorporated into membrane phospholipids, but there is also accumulating evidence of the relevance of this type of fatty acid in liver metabolism. In fact, it has been reported that DHA may have unique effects on hepatic gene expression [12]. Particularly the transcription of genes involved in the control of hepatic glycolysis and lipogenesis seems to be regulated by the function and/or physical interaction of DHA with special transcription factors, like PPARα, SREBP-1, ChREBP and MLX, and several signaling pathways, including AKT, ERK1/2, GSK3 and PKC [12]. These findings highlight that changes in DHA content may have a major impact on hepatic lipid and carbohydrate metabolism.

Besides these metabolic effects of DHA, some studies are highly suggestive that this n-3 PUFA may exert several anti-inflammatory actions, including the partial inhibition of leukocyte chemotaxis, adhesion molecule expression, adhesive interactions of leukocytes and endothelial cells, as well as the production and release of the most common proinflammatory cytokines (TNF-α, IL-1β and IL-6). These anti-inflammatory effects of DHA depend on its ability to alter cell membrane phospholipid composition, to disrupt lipid rafts and to hamper the transcriptional activity of transcription factor nuclear factor-κB, which controls the expression of proinflammatory cytokines [4]. The broad anti-inflammatory effects of DHA and other n-3 PUFAs are mediated by GPR120 [6]. DHA can activate GPR120 expression on macrophages causing a broad spectrum of anti-inflammatory effects, which in turn may result in insulin-sensitizing and antidiabetic effects in vivo [6]. Recently, Raptis et al. [13] demonstrated that GPR120 is also expressed by Kupffer cells, in which it plays a crucial role as a mediator of the beneficial effects of a commercial formulation of n-3 PUFA.

## Overview of Pediatric Nonalcoholic Fatty Liver Disease

In the last three decades, the prevalence of overweight/obesity in the pediatric population of industrialized countries has more than tripled, causing the onset of metabolic diseases – also in pediatric age – of diseases previously considered diseases of adults exclusively, such as diabetes mellitus type 2, cardiovascular diseases and the metabolic syndrome [9].

NAFLD now represents the most frequent cause of chronic liver disease in children and adolescents, which is a direct consequence of the worldwide annual increase in the number of obese children. However, the precise incidence and prevalence of NAFLD/nonalcoholic steatohepatitis (NASH) remain unknown since published data with long-term follow-up are scant [14]. NAFLD affects approximately 3–10% of the general pediatric population, and this percentage increases up to >70% in obese children [15].

NAFLD is a group of liver diseases ranging from simple fat accumulation in hepatocytes (>5%) to NASH, with various degrees of inflammation and fibrosis [8].

Many advances have been made in the last decade in the understanding of pathogenetic mechanisms of liver diseases. Previously, the so-called 'two-hit hypothesis' has been used to explain the NAFLD/NASH pathophysiology, in which liver fat accumulation (first hit) increases hepatic vulnerability to 'second hits' (insulin resistance and oxidative stress), causing disease progression. Actually, based on new discoveries, this model has been changed in a 'multiple-hit' hypothesis, in which a complex interplay between genetic, epigenetic and environmental factors is involved in the development and progression of pediatric NAFLD [16]. Recent studies have focused on the heritability of NAFLD, identifying single nucleotide polymorphisms in genes involved in lipid metabolism, oxidative stress and fibrogenesis associated with the severity of liver injury [17]. NAFLD is initially characterized by fat accumulation in hepatocytes, caused by increased delivery of free fatty acids to the liver, lipogenesis and insulin resistance. Liver steatosis worsens insulin resistance by interfering with phosphorylation of insulin receptor substrates [18]. These metabolic injuries predispose the liver cells to further liver damage derived from oxidative stress, mitochondrial dysfunction, proinflammatory cytokine imbalance and stellate cell activation, inducing the progression of liver disease to necroinflammation and fibrosis. Recent data demonstrated that, in the fibrogenetic process during NASH development, a central role is played by hepatic stellate/progenitor cells, which respond to oxidative stress with activation and proliferation causing a ductular reaction and fibrosis. Moreover, the increase in visceral fat is associated with a decrease in the release of insulin-sensitizing and anti-inflammatory cytokines, and an increase in the release of proinflammatory molecules. Therefore, based on recent discoveries, an intricate cross talk between hepatocytes, hepatic progenitor cells, gut cells and adipocytokines has been hypothesized [19].

The primary goal of treatment of pediatric NAFLD is represented by the reversion up to full recovery of liver damage. The first line of treatment of NAFLD remains weight loss through diet and regular physical activity. Unfortunately, several international studies showed that changes in lifestyle are very difficult to obtain in children with scarce results on weight loss and metabolic comorbidities. To date, no guideline for pharmacological therapy of fatty liver disease is available. The majority of drugs tested in randomized clinical trials, such as metformin, vitamin E and ursodeoxycholic acid, have yielded disappointing results in improving liver damage [20].

## Docosahexaenoic Acid and Pediatric Nonalcoholic Fatty Liver Disease

There is consensus on the treatment of pediatric NAFLD to date. However, improved lifestyle and reduction in body weight represent the first-line steps in order to improve the hepatic steatosis and to avoid the progression toward liver fibrosis. Furthermore, a diet high in monounsaturated fatty acids and PUFAs (n-3 and n-6 PUFAs) seems beneficial.

Supplementation with n-3 and n-6 PUFAs in patients affected by NAFLD was performed. A recent meta-analysis [7] described the beneficial effects of n-3 supplementation given to adults affected by NAFLD at a dose of at least 0.83 g/day. As a result of this integration, a decreased level of triglycerides and LDL and an increased level of HDL were obtained as well as a significant improvement in hepatic steatosis investigated by ultrasound (US). Here, we focused on the few studies that reported the effects of DHA in children with NAFLD (table 1).

Nobili et al. [21] performed the first randomized controlled trial in a pediatric population. In this trial, 60 children affected by NAFLD were enrolled and randomized into three groups: the first received 250 mg/day of DHA, the second received 500 mg/day of DHA and the third received the placebo. After 6 months of DHA (n-3) supplementation, meaningful reductions in triglyceride levels and insulin resistance

**Table 1.** Randomized controlled trials on DHA in pediatric NAFLD

| Authors | Year | Patients | DHA, mg/day | Results |
|---|---|---|---|---|
| Nobili et al. [21] | 2011 | 60 children with US-proven NAFLD | 250–500 | After 6 months: improvement triglycerides, insulin resistance and hepatic steatosis (US) |
| Nobili et al. [22] | 2013 | 60 children with US-proven NAFLD | 250–500 | After 24 months: improvement triglycerides, insulin resistance and hepatic steatosis (US) |
| Jaczyk et al. [23] | 2013 | 76 children with US-proven NAFLD | 830 | After 6 months: improvement ALT (>0.3 ULN) and hepatic steatosis (US) |
| Nobili et al. [24] | 2014 | 20 children with biopsy-proven NAFLD | 250–500 | After 18 months: improvement triglycerides, insulin resistance TNF-α, IL-6 and steatosis, ballooning, lobular inflammation |

were noticed; in addition, a significant improvement of hepatic steatosis was noted by US. Moreover, both DHA administrations (250 and 500 mg/day) appear to be equally effective in reducing hepatic steatosis.

The same results on metabolic parameters were obtained after 24 months of DHA supplementation, with no significant effect on body mass index and alanine transaminase (ALT) levels [22].

In contrast to this last observation, Jaczyk et al. [23] disclosed a lower ALT level (>0.3 ULN) after supplementation of n-3 PUFAs for 24 weeks in their randomized controlled trial conducted in 76 children (6–19 years old); this finding was associated with a beneficial effect on metabolic parameters and with an improvement of liver steatosis.

Subsequently, Nobili et al. [24] investigated the effect of 18 months of DHA supplementation on hepatic damage by histological evaluation. The study showed a beneficial effect of DHA on metabolic parameters that also concerned the stage of steatosis, with a reduction in ballooning and lobular inflammation on histologic examination, but no effect on fibrosis. A significant reduction in serum levels of proinflammatory cytokines (TNF-α and IL-6) was also demonstrated.

Supplementation with DHA seems to have both a strong anti-inflammatory action and a beneficial effect on insulin sensitivity; it also reduces the inflammatory macrophage pool acting on receptor GPR120. Therefore, GRP120 seems to play a key role in the inflammatory response in hepatocytes and progenitor cell activation and survival as well as in insulin resistance (fig. 1).

In the last years, the role of genetic factors in the development of NAFLD was defined. A study by Nobili et al. [25] showed that DHA supplementation induces

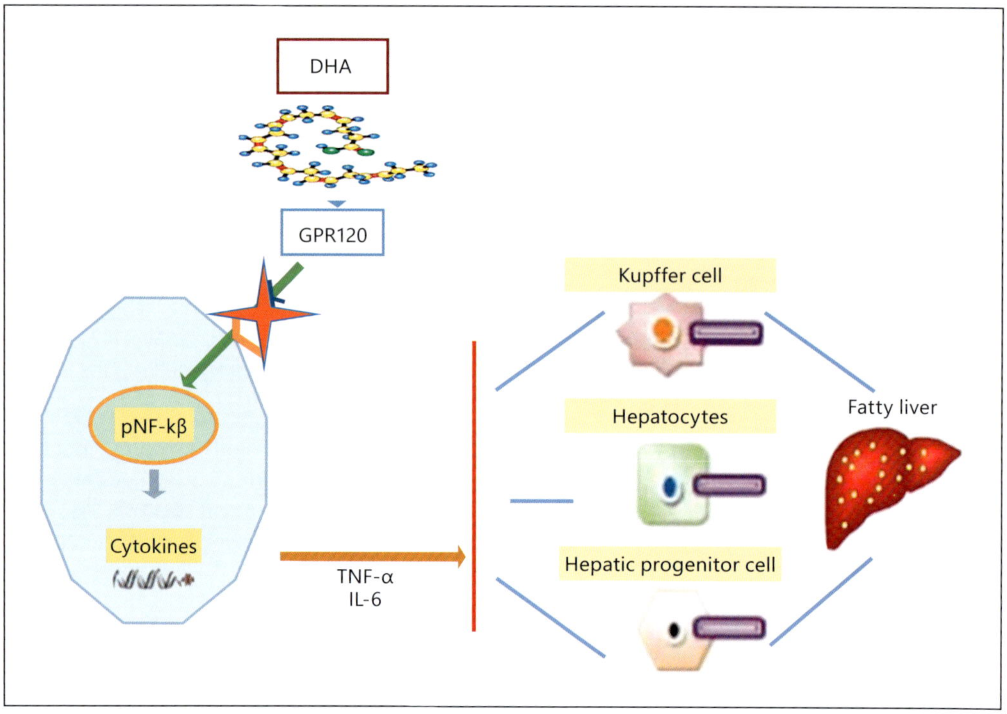


**Fig. 1.** Mechanism for beneficial effects of DHA (modified from Nobili et al. [27]).

different responses depending on patatin-like phospholipase-containing domain 3 (PNPLA3) genetic polymorphisms. The presence of allele 148M of PNPLA3 prevents an optimal response to treatment with DHA, unlike the presence of allele 148I [25]. In view of these results, Marzuillo et al. [26] investigated the role of genetic polymorphisms and GRP120 in the progression of liver injury in NAFLD. The study showed that the presence of the allele R270H of GRP120 is associated with abnormal serum ALT level. R270H increases susceptibility to develop NASH and counteracts the anti-inflammatory activity of DHA. In addition, there could be a significant interaction between PNPLA3 and GRP120. The presence of GPR120 R270H and I148M of PNPLA3 was associated with a higher risk of ALT level increase and appeared to promote NASH.

## Conclusions

Supplementation with DHA seems to be of proven efficacy in the prevention and treatment of cardiovascular diseases, dyslipidemia as well as in the metabolic syndrome. The reduction in the GRP120 signal, due to a poor n-3 PUFA diet as well as the presence of predisposing genetic factors, may induce the activation of Kupffer cells and inflammation during NAFLD. Therefore, it is conceivable that DHA/GRP120 may play a pivotal role in slowing the progression of liver damage in patients with NAFLD. However, as the beneficial effects of DHA could depend on genetic factors, continued research is required in order to establish the optimal regimen of DHA in the management and prevention of the metabolic syndrome.

## References


1 Burri L, Hoem N, Banni S, Berge K: Marine omega-3 phospholipids: metabolism and biological activities. Int J Mol Sci 2012;13:15401–15419.

2 Simopoulos AP: The importance of the ratio of omega-6/omega-3 essential fatty acids. Biomed Pharmacother 2002;56:365–379.

3 Kwak SM, Myung SK, Lee YJ, Seo HG: Efficacy of omega-3 fatty acid supplements (eicosapentaenoic acid and docosahexaenoic acid) in the secondary prevention of cardiovascular disease: a meta-analysis of randomized, double-blind, placebo-controlled trials. Arch Intern Med 2012;172:686–694.

4 Calder PC: Omega-3 polyunsaturated fatty acids and inflammatory processes: nutrition or pharmacology? Br J Clin Pharmacol 2013;75:645–662.

5 Pinel A, Morio-Liondore B, Capel F: n-3 polyunsaturated fatty acids modulate metabolism of insulin-sensitive tissues: implication for the prevention of type 2 diabetes. J Physiol Biochem 2014;70:647–658.

6 Oh DY, Talukdar S, Bae EJ, Imamura T, Morinaga H, Fan W, Li P, Lu WJ, Watkins SM, Olefsky JM: GPR120 is an omega-3 fatty acid receptor mediating potent anti-inflammatory and insulin-sensitizing effects. Cell 2010;142:687–698.

7 Parker HM, Johnson NA, Burdon CA, Cohn JS, O'Connor HT, George J: Omega-3 supplementation and non-alcoholic fatty liver disease: a systematic review and meta-analysis. J Hepatol 2012;56:944–951.

8 Brunt EM: Nonalcoholic fatty liver disease: what the pathologist can tell the clinician. Dig Dis 2012; 30(suppl 1):61–68.

9 Alisi A, Manco M, Vania A, Nobili V: Pediatric nonalcoholic fatty liver disease in 2009. J Pediatr 2009; 155:469–474.

10 Vernon G, Baranova A, Younossi ZM: Systematic review: the epidemiology and natural history of nonalcoholic fatty liver disease and non-alcoholic steatohepatitis in adults. Aliment Pharmacol Ther 2011; 34:274–285.

11 Stillwell W, Wassall SR: Docosahexaenoic acid: membrane properties of a unique fatty acid. Chem Phys Lipids 2003;126:1–27.

12 Jump DB, Botolin D, Wang Y, Xu J, Demeure O, Christian B: Docosahexaenoic acid (DHA) and hepatic gene transcription. Chem Phys Lipids 2008; 153:3–13.

13 Raptis DA, Limani P, Jang JH, Ungethüm U, Tschuor C, Graf R, Humar B, Clavien PA: GPR120 on Kupffer cells mediates hepatoprotective effects of ω3-fatty acids. J Hepatol 2014;60:625–632.

14 Feldstein AE, Charatcharoenwitthaya P, Treeprasertsuk S, Benson JT, Enders FB, Angulo P: The natural history of nonalcoholic fatty liver disease in children: a follow-up study for up to 20 years. Gut 2009;58: 1538–1544.

15 Schwimmer JB, Deutsch R, Kahen T, Lavine JE, Stanley C, Behling C: Prevalence of fatty liver in children and adolescents. Pediatrics 2006;118:1388–1393.

16 Alisi A, Cianfarani S, Manco M, Agostoni C, Nobili V: Non-alcoholic fatty liver disease and metabolic syndrome in adolescents: pathogenetic role of genetic background and intrauterine environment. Ann Med 2012;44:29–40.

17 Nobili V, Donati B, Panera N, Vongsakulyanon A, Alisi A, Dallapiccola B, Valenti L: A four-polymorphism risk score predicts steatohepatitis in children with non-alcoholic fatty liver disease. J Pediatr Gastroenterol Nutr 2014;58:632–636.

18 Samuel VT, Liu ZX, Qu X, Elder BD, Bilz S, Befroy D, Romanelli AJ, Shulman GI: Mechanism of hepatic insulin resistance in non-alcoholic fatty liver disease. J Biol Chem 2004;279:32345–32353.

19 Nobili V, Svegliati-Baroni G, Alisi A, Miele L, Valenti L, Vajro P: A 360-degree overview of paediatric NAFLD: recent insights. J Hepatol 2013;58:1218–1229.

20 Della Corte C, Liccardo D, Ferrari F, Alisi A, Nobili V: Current pharmacotherapy for treating pediatric nonalcoholic fatty liver disease. Expert Opin Pharmacother 2014;15:2501–2511.

21 Nobili V, Bedogni G, Alisi A, Pietrobattista A, Risé P, Galli C, Agostoni C: Docosahexaenoic acid supplementation decreases liver fat content in children with non-alcoholic fatty liver disease: double blind randomized controlled clinical trial. Arch Child 2011;96:350–353.

22 Nobili V, Alisi A, Della Corte C, Risé P, Galli C, Agostoni C, Bedogni G: Docosahexaenoic acid for the treatment of fatty liver: randomized controlled trial in children. Nutr Metab Cardiovasc Dis 2013; 23:1066–1070.

23 Jaczyk W, Socha P, Lebensztejn D, Wierzbicka A, Mazur A, Neuhoff-Murawska J, Matusik P: Omega-3 fatty acid for treatment of non-alcoholic fatty liver disease: design and rationale of randomized controlled trial. BMC Pediatr 2013;23:13–85.

24 Nobili V, Carpino G, Alisi A, De Vito R, Franchitto A, Alpini G, Onori P, Gaudio E: Role of docosahexaenoic acid treatment in improving liver histology in pediatric nonalcoholic fatty liver disease. PLoS One 2014;9:e88005.

25 Nobili V, Bedogni G, Donati B, Alisi A, Valenti L: The I148M variant of PNPLA3 reduces the response to docosahexaenoic acid in children with non-alcoholic fatty liver disease. J Med Food 2013;16:957–960.

26 Marzuillo P, Grandone A, Conte M, Capuano F, Cirillo G, Di Sessa A, Umano GR, Romano R, Perrone L, del Giudice EM: Novel association between a nonsynonymous variant (R207H) of the G-protein-coupled receptor 120 and liver injury in children and adolescents with obesity. J Pediatr Gastroenterol Nutr 2014;59:472–475.

27 Nobili V, Alkhouri N, Alisi A, Della Corte C, Fitzpatrick E, Raponi M, Dhawan A: Nonalcoholic fatty liver disease: a challenge for pediatricians. JAMA Pediatr 2015;169:170–176.

Prof. Valerio Nobili
Hepato-Metabolic Disease Unit
Bambino Gesù Children's Hospital
IRCCS, Piazza Sant'Onofrio 4, IT–00165 Rome (Italy)
E-Mail nobili66@yahoo.it

Cappa M, Cianfarani S, Ghizzoni L, Loche S, Maghnie M (eds): Advanced Therapies in Pediatric Endocrinology and Diabetology. Endocr Dev. Basel, Karger, 2016, vol 30, pp 37–41 (DOI: 10.1159/000439326)

# Noninvasive Prenatal Diagnosis of Congenital Adrenal Hyperplasia

Ahmed Khattab[a] · Tony Yuen[a] · Li Sun[a] · Mabel Yau[a] · Ariella Barhan[a] · Mone Zaidi[a] · Y.M. Dennis Lo[b] · Maria I. New[a]

[a]Departments of Pediatrics and Medicine, Icahn School of Medicine at Mount Sinai, New York, N.Y., USA; [b]Department of Chemical Pathology, The Chinese University of Hong Kong, Hong Kong, SAR, China

**Abstract**

A major hallmark of classical congenital adrenal hyperplasia (CAH) is genital ambiguity noted at birth in affected females, which leads to psychological and psychosexual issues in adult life. Attempts to correct genital ambiguity through surgical intervention have been partially successful. Fetal hyperandrogenemia and genital ambiguity have been shown to be preventable by prenatal administration of low-dose dexamethasone initiated before the 9th week of gestation. In 7 of 8 at-risk pregnancies, the unaffected fetus is unnecessarily exposed to dexamethasone for weeks until the diagnosis of classical CAH is ruled out by invasive procedures. This therapeutic dilemma calls for early prenatal diagnosis so that dexamethasone treatment can be directed to affected female fetuses only. We describe the utilization of cell-free fetal DNA in mothers carrying at-risk fetuses as early as 6 gestational weeks by targeted massively parallel sequencing of the genomic region including and flanking the CYP21A2 gene. Our highly personalized and innovative approach should permit the diagnosis of CAH before genital development begins, therefore restricting the purposeful administration of dexamethasone to mothers carrying affected females. 

Congenital adrenal hyperplasia (CAH) is the most prevalent rare monogenic disorder with an overall incidence of 1 in 15,000 live births [1]. Around 90% of CAH cases are due to mutations in the *CYP21A2* gene, all of which reduce the activity of the enzyme 21-hydroxylase, but to varying extents. Three clinical phenotypes thus arise, namely salt wasting, simple virilizing (the two grouped as classical CAH) and nonclassical CAH. About 150 disease-causing *CYP21A2* mutations have been identified.

We recently completed a full clinical characterization of genotype-phenotype concordance in 1,507 families [2]. We also used computational modeling to predict the functional loss that each mutation induces by altering the conformation of 21-hydroxylase [3].

A major hallmark of classical CAH is genital ambiguity noted at birth in affected females; this leads to psychological and psychosexual issues in adult life. Attempts to correct genital ambiguity through surgical intervention have been successful only in part, as these procedures can result in urinary incontinence and sexual dysfunction [4–6].

Forest et al. [7, 8] first showed that fetal hyperandrogenemia and genital ambiguity are preventable by low-dose dexamethasone (20 μg/kg/day to a maximum dose of 1.5 mg/day) given orally to pregnant at-risk mothers. Without binding to corticosteroid-binding globulin or being metabolized by placental 11β-hydroxysteroid dehydrogenase, dexamethasone crosses the placenta to enter the fetus. Here, it suppresses androgen production to prevent in utero virilization and genital ambiguity. Prenatal dexamethasone therapy must be initiated before the 9th week of gestation to coincide with the onset of urogenital development. However, a definitive genetic diagnosis of CAH can only be made by chorionic villus sampling (CVS) or amniocentesis around week 12 or 14, respectively. Therefore, even while male and unaffected female fetuses will not benefit from prenatal dexamethasone, we must treat *all* mothers with at-risk fetuses before invasive diagnostic testing reveals fetal sex and genetic diagnosis. This means that 7 of 8 pregnant mothers are exposed to dexamethasone without benefit, with half of their fetuses being males and three quarters of the females being unaffected. This therapeutic dilemma calls for *early* prenatal diagnosis so that dexamethasone treatment can be directed to affected female fetuses only.

In 1997, our collaborator, Prof. Y.M. Dennis Lo, reported the successful detection of cell-free fetal DNA in maternal plasma – this ushered new possibilities for the noninvasive prenatal diagnosis of monogenic disorders, including CAH [9]. Before this discovery, a noninvasive prenatal diagnosis was possible only by isolating nucleated fetal cells in the maternal circulation. However, these cells are known to remain in the maternal circulation, thus potentially confounding prenatal genetic analysis in subsequent pregnancies [10, 11]. In contrast, cell-free fetal DNA disappears from the maternal circulation within 24 h after birth. A pregnancy under study thus does not capture cell-free fetal DNA from a former pregnancy [12].

In a recent collaborative study with Prof. Lo, we utilized cell-free fetal DNA in ~3.6 ml of plasma drawn from 14 mothers carrying at-risk fetuses as early as 6 gestational weeks (fig. 1) [13]. Unfortunately, simple PCR, otherwise used for routine genetic testing, cannot be used on these plasma samples due to interference by vast amounts of maternal DNA and because fetal DNA is fragmented. Further, in the case of CAH, long-range PCR cannot be performed to differentiate mutations in *CYP21A2* (which we are looking for) from those in the homologous pseudogene *CYP21A1P*. We have therefore made the diagnosis of CAH by targeted massively parallel sequencing (MPS) of the genomic region including and flanking the *CYP21A2* gene. This innovative strategy of quantifying the amount of DNA inherited from the father and mother has allowed us to arrive at the allelic composition around the *CYP21A2* locus of the fetus.

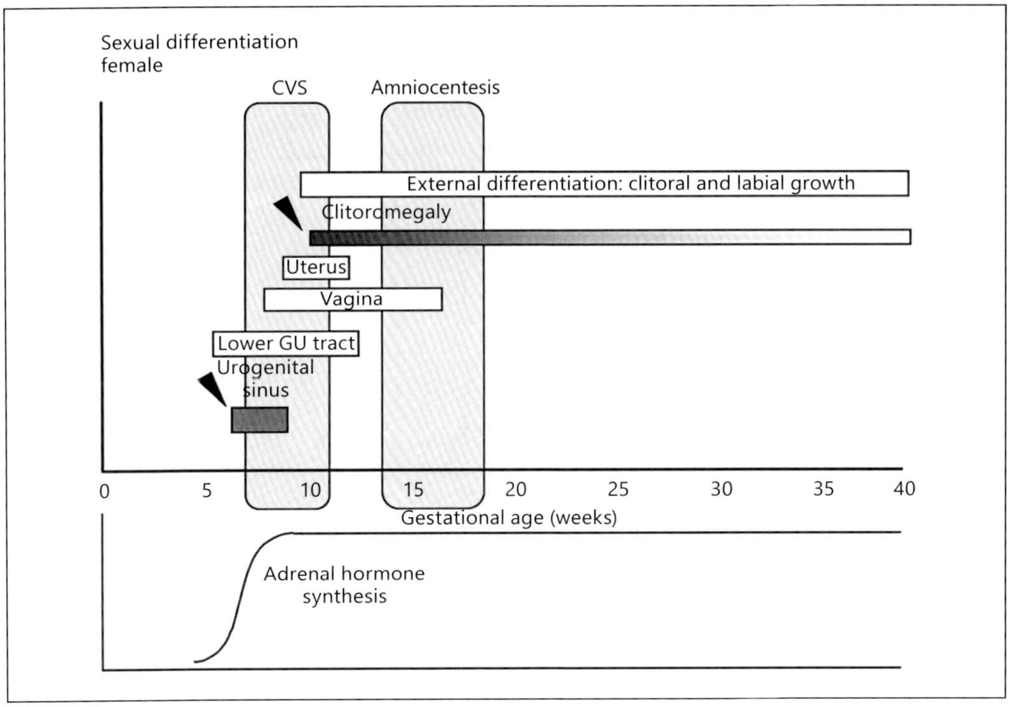


**Fig. 1.** Early prenatal diagnosis allows dexamethasone treatment to be directed to affected female fetuses only. GU = Genitourinary.

We noted 100% concordance between this technology and our standard invasive procedure in diagnosing CAH in all 14 cases [13].

The profound significance of our study stems from the fact that CAH owing to 21-hydroxylase deficiency is one of the few genetic disorders amenable to successful prenatal treatment. Our highly personalized and innovative approach should permit the diagnosis of CAH before genital development begins, therefore restricting the purposeful administration of dexamethasone to mothers carrying affected females [13]. In the future, our aim is to validate and utilize MPS for the genetic diagnosis of CAH before 9 weeks of gestation in the clinical setting.

We have also determined fetal sex by identifying fetus-derived chromosome Y sequences in maternal plasma by MPS [13]. In parallel, we also utilize PCR using an *SRY* probe, similarly to the approach used by Tardy-Guidollet et al. [14]. Results of the PCR, available within hours of fetal DNA isolation, can be used to eliminate unnecessary treatment of mothers carrying male fetuses. Furthermore, males affected with CAH are not normally diagnosed at birth as there is no genital ambiguity. Genotyping male fetuses, particularly those with severe salt-wasting mutations, should additionally prompt physicians to initiate immediate therapy at birth with glucocorticoids, mineralocorticoids and dietary salt to prevent adrenal crises and possible mortality. Early prenatal diagnosis will also allow ample time for parental

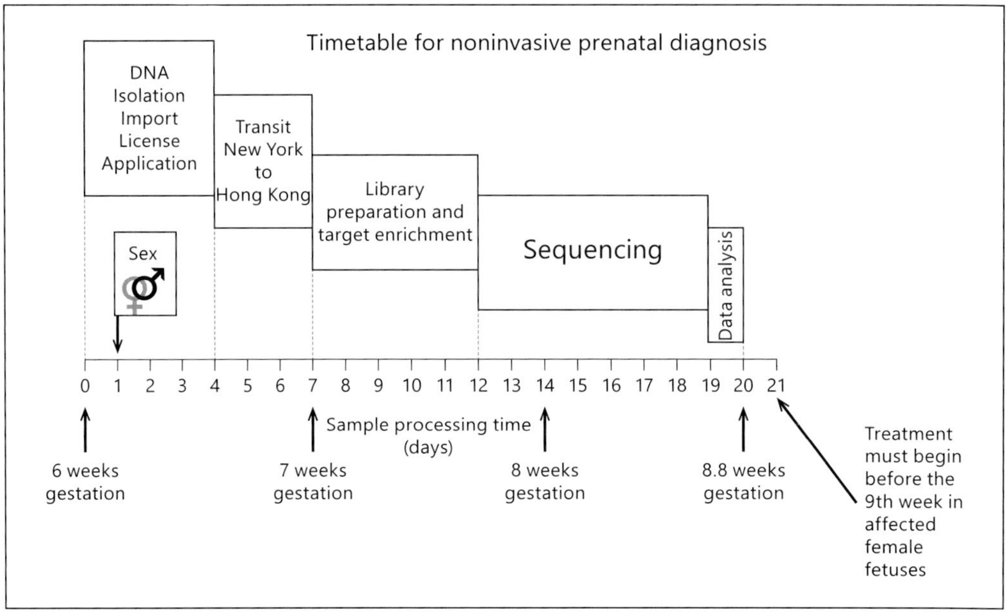


**Fig. 2.** This timetable is currently utilized owing to our collaboration with Prof. Lo in Hong Kong.

counseling regarding postnatal care of a newborn with severe life-threatening CAH (fig. 2).

*Significance.* Apart from the very specific advantages of early diagnosis in (a) personalizing the use of dexamethasone to prevent genital ambiguity in affected female fetuses, and (b) initiating early therapy to prevent morbidity and mortality in severe salt-wasting CAH, MPS-based testing holds promise for the early diagnosis of a variety of other monogenic disorders. Only few, including β-thalassemia [15], achondroplasia [16], and cystic fibrosis [17], have hitherto been tested noninvasively. However, it is needless to emphasize that while the risks associated with invasive procedures, such as pregnancy loss and spontaneous miscarriage [18], are low, they nonetheless remain clinically significant. More rarely, these procedures are associated with malformations, such as talipes and hemangiomas [18, 19]. Although amniocentesis and CVS are relatively safe, the significance of treating only affected females with dexamethasone remains paramount. Remote regions of developing countries, where sterile facilities for CVS and amniocentesis are unavailable, could potentially benefit from maternal plasma-based testing. A blood sample from a pregnant mother, which does not require sterile facilities, could be transported to specialized centers for MPS and haplotype linkage analysis. We expect that, over time, with the anticipated reduction in next-generation sequencing costs, noninvasive prenatal diagnosis will become the method of choice worldwide for a whole array of monogenic disorders.

## References


1 New MI, Lekarev O, Mancenido D, Parsa A, Yuen T: Congenital adrenal hyperplasia owing to 21-hydroxylase deficiency; in New MI, Lekarev O, Parsa A, Yuen TT, O'Malley BW, Hammer GD (eds): Genetic Steroid Disorders. San Diego, Academic Press, 2014, chapt 3A, pp 29–51.
2 New MI, Abraham M, Gonzalez B, Dumic M, Razzaghy-Azar M, Chitayat D, et al: Genotype-phenotype correlation in 1,507 families with congenital adrenal hyperplasia owing to 21-hydroxylase deficiency. Proc Natl Acad Sci U S A 2013;110:2611–2616.
3 Haider S, Islam B, D'Atri V, Sgobba M, Poojari C, Sun L, et al: Structure-phenotype correlations of human CYP21A2 mutations in congenital adrenal hyperplasia. Proc Natl Acad Sci U S A 2013;110:2605–2610.
4 Nordenstrom A, Frisen L, Falhammar H, Filipsson H, Holmdahl G, Janson PO, et al: Sexual function and surgical outcome in women with congenital adrenal hyperplasia due to CYP21A2 deficiency: clinical perspective and the patients' perception. J Clin Endocrinol Metab 2010;95:3633–3640.
5 Crouch NS, Liao LM, Woodhouse CR, Conway GS, Creighton SM: Sexual function and genital sensitivity following feminizing genitoplasty for congenital adrenal hyperplasia. J Urol 2008;179:634–638.
6 Crouch NS, Minto CL, Laio LM, Woodhouse CR, Creighton SM: Genital sensation after feminizing genitoplasty for congenital adrenal hyperplasia: a pilot study. BJU Int 2004;93:135–138.
7 Forest MG, Betuel H, David M: Prenatal treatment in congenital adrenal hyperplasia due to 21-hydroxylase deficiency: up-date 88 of the French multicentric study. Endocr Res 1989;15:277–301.
8 Forest MG, David M, Morel Y: Prenatal diagnosis and treatment of 21-hydroxylase deficiency. J Steroid Biochem Mol Biol 1993;45:75–82.
9 Lo YM, Corbetta N, Chamberlain PF, Rai V, Sargent IL, Redman CW, et al: Presence of fetal DNA in maternal plasma and serum. Lancet 1997;350:485–487.
10 Lo YM: Fetal DNA in maternal plasma: biology and diagnostic applications. Clin Chem 2000;46:1903–1906.
11 Bianchi DW, Zickwolf GK, Weil GJ, Sylvester S, DeMaria MA: Male fetal progenitor cells persist in maternal blood for as long as 27 years postpartum. Proc Natl Acad Sci U S A 1996;93:705–708.
12 Lo YM, Zhang J, Leung TN, Lau TK, Chang AM, Hjelm NM: Rapid clearance of fetal DNA from maternal plasma. Am J Hum Genet 1999;64:218–224.
13 New MI, Tong YK, Yuen T, Jiang P, Pina C, Chan KC, et al: Noninvasive prenatal diagnosis of congenital adrenal hyperplasia using cell-free fetal DNA in maternal plasma. J Clin Endocrinol Metab 2014;99:E1022–E1030.
14 Tardy-Guidollet V, Menassa R, Costa JM, David M, Bouvattier-Morel C, Baumann C, et al: New management strategy of pregnancies at risk of congenital adrenal hyperplasia using fetal sex determination in maternal serum: French cohort of 258 cases (2002–2011). J Clin Endocrinol Metab 2014;99:1180–1188.
15 Lun FM, Tsui NB, Chan KC, Leung TY, Lau TK, Charoenkwan P, et al: Noninvasive prenatal diagnosis of monogenic diseases by digital size selection and relative mutation dosage on DNA in maternal plasma. Proc Natl Acad Sci U S A 2008;105:19920–19925.
16 Saito H, Sekizawa A, Morimoto T, Suzuki M, Yanaihara T: Prenatal DNA diagnosis of a single-gene disorder from maternal plasma. Lancet 2000;356:1170.
17 Gonzalez-Gonzalez MC, Garcia-Hoyos M, Trujillo MJ, Rodriguez de Alba M, Lorda-Sanchez I, Diaz-Recasens J, et al: Prenatal detection of a cystic fibrosis mutation in fetal DNA from maternal plasma. Prenat Diagn 2002;22:946–948.
18 Alfirevic Z, Sundberg K, Brigham S: Amniocentesis and chorionic villus sampling for prenatal diagnosis. Cochrane Database Syst Rev 2003;3:CD003252.
19 Bauland CG, Smit JM, Scheffers SM, Bartels RH, van den Berg P, Zeebregts CJ, et al: Similar risk for hemangiomas after amniocentesis and transabdominal chorionic villus sampling. J Obstet Gynaecol Res 2012;38:371–375.



Maria I. New, MD
Department of Pediatrics, Room 419
Icahn School of Medicine at Mount Sinai, Annex Building
1249 5th Avenue, New York, NY 10029 (USA)
E-Mail maria.new@mssm.edu

Cappa M, Cianfarani S, Ghizzoni L, Loche S, Maghnie M (eds): Advanced Therapies in Pediatric Endocrinology and Diabetology. Endocr Dev. Basel, Karger, 2016, vol 30, pp 42–53 (DOI: 10.1159/000439329)

# Recent Advances in Hydrocortisone Replacement Treatment

Ashwini Mallappa[a] · Miguel Debono[b]

[a]Clinical Center, National Institutes of Health, Bethesda, Md., USA; [b]Academic Unit of Endocrinology, The Medical School, University of Sheffield, Sheffield, UK

**Abstract**

Since the first use of cortisone in patients around 65 years ago, the use of synthetic glucocorticoids has made a crucial impact on the treatment of several diseases in medicine. Although significant reductions in morbidity and mortality have occurred in patients suffering from cortisol deficiency, conventional hydrocortisone replacement treatment is still inadequate. A major limitation is that it fails to replace cortisol in a physiological manner. Cortisol has a distinct circadian rhythm and acts as a secondary messenger synchronizing the central to peripheral clocks, hence playing a key role in biological processes and the circadian timing system. Circadian misalignment has been associated with ill-health and so nonphysiological glucocorticoid treatment could explain the increased mortality rate, poor quality of life and metabolic complications in patients suffering from adrenal insufficiency. Attempts at replacing cortisol in a physiological manner have shown significant progress in the past decade with the development of modified-release formulations of hydrocortisone (Chronocort® and Plenadren®) and continuous subcutaneous hydrocortisone infusions. Initial studies investigating the use of these replacement regimens are promising, demonstrating both clinical and biochemical improvement. Larger studies are needed to determine whether this novel approach enhances long-term outcomes in both children and adults with cortisol deficiency.


Published by S. Karger AG, Basel.

Akin to several plant and animal species, important biological processes in humans exhibit circadian rhythmicity. The circadian timing system is controlled by the central 'master pacemaker' clock located in the hypothalamic suprachiasmatic nucleus of the human brain. This communicates with peripheral clocks in different cells, tissues and organs via neural and hormone signals. The major external factor (environmental cue) entraining this system is the light/dark cycle, whereas feeding and body temperature are implicated in the entrainment of peripheral pacemakers [1].

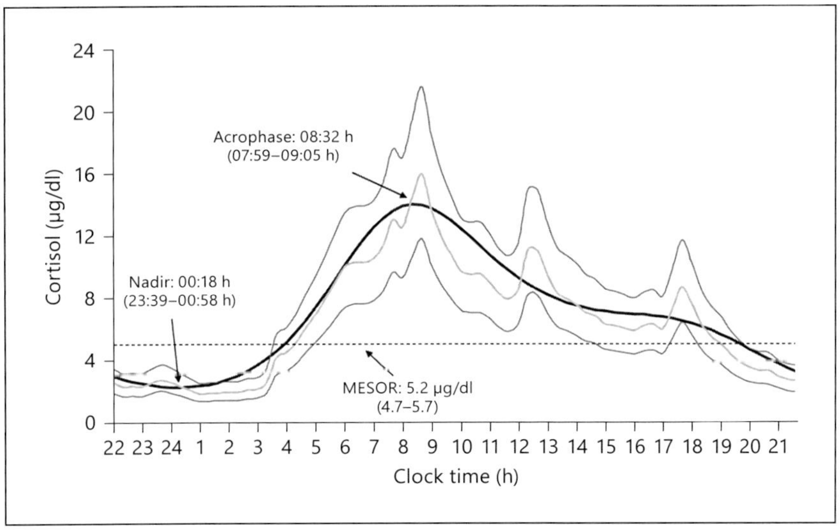


**Fig. 1.** Physiological circadian cortisol rhythm showing that cortisol levels begin to rise between 02:00 and 04:00 h, peak on awakening and then decline through the day reaching the nadir at around midnight (republished with permission from the Endocrine Society [2]).

Regulated by the hypothalamic-pituitary-adrenal axis, cortisol exhibits a distinct circadian rhythm overlying a dynamic ultradian rhythm. Signals from the central clock (suprachiasmatic nucleus) are transmitted to the hypothalamic paraventricular nucleus initiating the circadian release of corticotrophin-releasing hormone, which in turn drives the circadian rhythmicity of adrenocorticotropic hormone (ACTH) stimulating cortisol secretion in a distinctive pattern. Cortisol levels begin to rise between 02:00 and 04:00 h, peaking on awakening and then decline through the day, reaching the nadir at around midnight (fig. 1) [2]. Evidence suggests that glucocorticoids are likely secondary messengers synchronizing the central to peripheral clocks [3, 4].

Cortisol rhythmicity is altered in disease states such as adrenal insufficiency (AI), depression and obstructive sleep apnea, individuals on an alternative work schedule (night-shift workers) and in people travelling across time zones (jet lag). Shift work has been associated with higher cortisol awakening responses, increased 24-hour cortisol exposure and a slower cortisol decline over the day [5]. Jet lag results in temporal disorganization of both ACTH and cortisol secretion [6]. Sleeping and eating 12 h out of phase, a situation analogous acutely to jet lag and chronically to shift work, has been shown to result in complete inversion of the cortisol rhythm with high cortisol levels before sleeping potentially contributing to worsening insulin resistance and high glucose levels [7]. Such derangements are associated with fatigue, sleep disturbances and an increased risk of adverse cardiovascular and metabolic outcomes highlighting the importance of the cortisol rhythm to health.

## Problems in Adrenal Insufficiency – Why Could Physiological Replacement Enhance Management?

Individuals with AI irrespective of the etiology (primary, secondary or tertiary) require long-term glucocorticoid replacement therapy. Availability of glucocorticoid preparations in the early 1950s dramatically changed the management of AI reducing morbidity and mortality. Nonetheless, patients with AI have a more than two-fold mortality risk mainly secondary to cardiovascular diseases, infections and cancer. Patients with autoimmune polyendocrine syndrome type 1 may have an even higher mortality (standardized mortality ratio 4.6, 95% CI 3.5–6%) [8]. Several reports have documented that patients with AI have impaired quality of life (QOL), sleep problems and an increased risk of cardiovascular, metabolic and osteoporosis outcomes [9–12]. The administration of nonphysiological glucocorticoid replacement could be an important contributor to these problems. It has been shown that the circadian variation in serum cortisol determines the circadian rhythm of osteocalcin [13] and that of insulin resistance [14]. Supranormal cortisol levels in the morning are associated with periods of insulin resistance starting around 4–6 h later and persisting for >16 h [14]. The early-morning rise in cortisol on the other hand stimulates gluconeogenesis resulting in higher fasting and postprandial glucose levels, and also induces lipolysis, ketogenesis and proteolysis to produce metabolic body fuels that may be important in sustaining everyday activities preventing fatigue [15]. When patients with AI were administered a modified-release formulation of prednisone in the evening, this decreased complaints of fatigue when compared to morning conventional prednisolone treatment [16]. In addition, in children with ACTH and growth hormone (GH) deficiency, nocturnal hypoglycemia detected by continuous glucose monitoring was frequent and this was related to lower hydrocortisone dosing [17]. These factors highlight the importance of the use of circadian treatment in patients with AI. In addition, mortality in patients with secondary AI is related to higher weight-adjusted and absolute hydrocortisone doses with hazard ratios for mortality of 4.56 (≥0.35 mg/kg) and 4 (≥30 mg) [18]. A worse health status is also associated with hydrocortisone doses >30 mg/day, and with respect to well-being and daily performance, thrice daily intake, the commonly recommended regime in most centers, is not always superior to twice daily treatment [19].

## Problems in Congenital Adrenal Hyperplasia – Managing Androgen Excess with Avoidance of Iatrogenic Glucocorticoid Excess

Individuals affected by congenital adrenal hyperplasia (CAH) have a defect in the cortisol biosynthesis pathway. CAH due to 21-hydroxylase enzyme deficiency (accounts for >95% of cases) is the most common form, which is characterized not only by cortisol and aldosterone deficiency but also by androgen excess. With the introduction of cortisone treatment and the incorporation of newborn screening in many countries from the 1990s for this potentially fatal disease, CAH patients are surviving into adulthood.

Management goals in CAH aim to replace the deficient hormones and control the excess androgens by addressing the overnight rise in ACTH, the driving factor. These management goals need to be achieved meticulously as suppression of androgens often requires supraphysiological doses of glucocorticoids running the risk of overtreatment and its associated comorbidities. Conversely, hyperandrogenism results in precocious puberty in children, hirsutism in females and infertility in both sexes. Recent Endocrine Society guidelines recommend thrice-daily hydrocortisone therapy at doses of 10–15 $mg/m^2/day$ for growing children [20]. On achieving adult height, children can be transitioned to longer-acting preparations. There are no such standard replacement guidelines for the management of adults with CAH. Several different regimens of short, intermediate or long-acting glucocorticoid regimens alone or in combination are used in clinical practice based on individual needs.

Large-cohort studies document metabolic abnormalities in CAH patients. The investigators of the CaHASE study conducted in the UK reported that in their cohort of 203 adults with CAH, 41% were found to be obese, 29% with insulin resistance, 46% with high cholesterol levels and close to 50% of patients with osteopenia or osteoporosis [21]. CAH patients also have impaired health-related QOL. Though patients were on several different glucocorticoid treatment regimens in the CaHASE cohort (26% on hydrocortisone, 43% on prednisolone, 18% on dexamethasone and 10% on a combination), disease control was highly variable. Only 36% of patients had normal androgen (androstenedione) levels; 38% had suppressed androgens indicating glucocorticoid overtreatment [21]. Similar results were seen in a US cohort (n = 244) which included children and adults [22].

Longer-acting formulations are commonly prescribed to increase compliance and/or to address disease complications such as adrenal rest tissue; these formulations (prednisolone and dexamethasone) are associated with increased adiposity, insulin resistance and impaired QOL, and thus a suboptimal treatment option [23].

Management of CAH in adolescence has unique challenges given the physiological changes that occur during this period with respect to cortisol metabolism [24]. Activation of the hypothalamic-pituitary-gonadal axis leads to increased levels of GH and insulin-like growth factor-1 which in turn increase glomerular filtration rate and decrease 11β-hydroxysteroid dehydrogenase type 1 enzyme activity leading to increased cortisol clearance. Higher estrogen levels in puberty increase levels of cortisol-binding globulin, thus, further decreasing free cortisol levels. These physiological changes during the key period of development call for frequent monitoring and dose adjustments. Increasing hydrocortisone dose frequency may be required but is not a practical solution given fluctuating compliance commonly seen in adolescents [25].

Management of CAH has specific challenges depending on individual factors. Clearly, current available regimens are suboptimal as they fail to simulate the physiological cortisol rhythm and fall short of addressing the disease-associated comorbidities, and contribute to adverse metabolic and impaired QOL outcomes in this patient population.

#### Current Hydrocortisone Treatment Regimens – Pitfalls and Inadequacies

Glucocorticoid replacement in AI is inadequate [26]. There is wide variation in hydrocortisone treatment regimens used in the management of AI. In a seminal pharmacokinetic study by Simon et al. [27], 13 different regimens were used by 50 different patients and, by using a cortisol day curve in patients on doses varying between 15 and 50 mg (mean dose 25 mg), 79, 55 and 45% were out of physiological range at 08:00, 16:00 and 24:00 h. The best regimen to reproduce physiological levels was found to be the 10-mg (07:30 h) + 5-mg (12:00 h) + 5-mg (16:30 h) regimen. But even using this regimen, about 54, 44 and 32% of patients will either be over- or undertreated at 08:00, 16:00 and 24:00 h, respectively. This highlights the challenges physicians face to try and approximate physiological cortisol levels using conventional hydrocortisone. Cortisol levels may climb to supraphysiological values minutes after dose administration, are below normal values before the next dose, and the early morning rise in cortisol is not produced. In addition, studies of the pharmacokinetics of hydrocortisone reveal wide interindividual variability in different parameters. After 10–20 mg of oral hydrocortisone, $C_{max}$ varied between 422 and 1,554 nmol/l and area under the curve (AUC) ranged between 1,081 and 5,471 nmol h/l in patients suffering from AI [28]. A number of factors could account for this variability, including different rates of absorption related to food intake, interactions with drugs that influence the cytochrome $P_{450}$-dependent pathway, binding of cortisol-binding globulin, volume distribution and hydrocortisone sensitivity, metabolism and excretion. Unfortunately, no standard glucocorticoid biomarkers are available to monitor treatment outcomes, so dose titration on an individual basis is not straightforward.

A recent consensus statement for the management of Addison's disease (AD) has recommended using a total daily dose of 15–25 mg of hydrocortisone, 25–37.5 mg of cortisone acetate as split dosing taken twice or three times or a total daily dose of 4–5 mg of prednisolone taken once or as split dosing (3 + 1 mg, 3 + 2 mg) twice daily [29]. Body surface area (expressed as $m^2$) dosing is recommended when treating children with recommendations to use a dose of 6–10 $mg/m^2$/day for AD management and 10–15 $mg/m^2$/day dosing for CAH management [20, 29]. In adults, weight-adjusted dosing has been investigated successfully. As shown in a study by Mah et al. [30], weight-adjusted dosing showed the least interindividual variability in $C_{max}$ and AUC when compared to body surface area-adjusted dosing and fixed dosing in addition to decreasing overexposure. The study further confirmed that 78% of the variability in AUC after 10 mg of hydrocortisone in the morning was explained by a serum cortisol level after 240 min, and this value could be used by physicians to adjust morning hydrocortisone doses using a nomogram. Other investigators have recommended other regimes, such as the use of four-times-daily dosing which when compared to twice-daily dosing gave higher 24-hour cortisol levels and lower ACTH exposure together with higher health-related QOL scores [31], which would be ideal but may compromise compliance. Other suggested schemes include the administration of hydrocortisone at 03:00 h in patients with CAH to control morning androgen levels. This technique was superior to giving higher or later evening doses but would be impractical to the patients [32].

The inadequacies of hydrocortisone replacement treatment in patients with AI and CAH are evident. Novel therapeutic strategies are essential, and this has led investigators to explore and investigate new treatments, one of which is circadian hydrocortisone replacement.

## Circadian Hydrocortisone Therapy – Recent Advancements

### *Oral Formulations*

To address the limitations of current conventional hydrocortisone preparations, newer formulations which are closer to and better at mimicking cortisol physiology are being evaluated. Plenadren®, marketed in Europe to be administered as a once-daily dose, is one such preparation. Plenadren® (ViroPharma, UK) is a dual-release hydrocortisone tablet with an immediate-release outer covering on a sustained-release core. Taken as first thing in the morning, Plenadren® 20 mg provides a clinically significant cortisol level (>200 nmol/l or >7 μg/dl) in approximately 20–40 min and peak levels (>400 nmol/l or 14.5 μg/dl) are seen within 1–2 h depending if the medication is taken in the fasting or nonfasting state, respectively. Serum cortisol levels remain >200 nmol/l for about 6 h after dosing and drop to <100 nmol/l (or 3.6 μg/dl) after around 10 h [33]. Use of Plenadren® in an open-label study in AD showed improvements in cardiovascular risk factors (weight, hemoglobin A1C and blood pressure) and significant improvements in fatigue but around 20% less cortisol exposure compared to thrice-daily hydrocortisone [34]. In the long term, the drug was well tolerated though there were 18.6 serious adverse events/100 patient-years of Plenadren® use [35]. This once-daily formulation does not provide the early morning physiological cortisol rise. Plenadren® also falls short of addressing the overnight increase in ACTH levels, which is the driving factor for high androgens in CAH patients.

Another oral formulation developed and studied by our group is Chronocort®. Previous studies showed that the use of a tablet-form modified-release formulation of hydrocortisone could approximate the cortisol circadian rhythm by reproducing the early morning rise in cortisol [2], and this pilot formulation achieved better control of morning androgens when compared to conventional hydrocortisone in patients with CAH [36]. Chronocort® showed encouraging results in a recent phase 2 clinical trial [37]. Chronocort® (Diurnal, UK) is a modified-release multiparticulate hydrocortisone capsule formulation developed using scalable technology. It has a pH-triggered enteric coat allowing dissolution in the small bowel providing delayed and sustained absorption kinetics [38]. In a 6-month study in 16 adults with CAH on several different glucocorticoid formulations at study entry, Chronocort® was initiated as 20 mg at 23:00 h and 10 mg at 07:00 h, and dose adjustments were made based on symptomatology and hormone status [androstenedione and 17-hydroxyprogesterone (17-OHP)]. The cortisol profile of Chronocort® in the patient population was similar to physiological cortisol secretion with an overnight cortisol rise and peak after awakening [2]. In comparison to conventional therapy, Chronocort® therapy at 6 months was effective in controlling the disease biomarkers, androstenedione and 17-OHP, with a lower hydrocortisone dose equivalency (conventional: 28 ± 11.8 mg/day vs. Chronocort® 25.9 ± 7.1 mg/day). Chronocort® resulted in lower 24-hour, morning (07:00–15:00 h) and afternoon (15:00–23:00 h) androstenedione AUC, and lower 24-hour and morning 17-OHP AUC (fig. 2). Chronocort® was overall well tolerated with no serious adverse events. In addition, there were positive changes in body composition (increase in lean mass/decrease in fat mass) and osteocalcin. We observed a decrease in bone mineral density, but this could be related to a reduction and better control of sex androgens. Further long-term studies with detailed assessment of bone mineral density, metabolic parameters, cardiovascular events and fracture risk are necessary.

*Continuous Subcutaneous Hydrocortisone Infusion Therapy*

Another novel route is use of a programmable pump for the delivery of cortisol as a continuous subcutaneous hydrocortisone infusion (CSHI) to approximate the physiological cortisol rhythm. This is being explored by our group and other researchers. At a minimum, a programmable pump can be set to deliver hydrocortisone in at least 24 different hourly rates. This unique feature of the programmable pump provides hope for replacing cortisol not only in a circadian pattern but also has potential for ultradian dosing [39]. In the last decade, promising results were seen from short-term open-label and proof-of-concept studies in patients with CAH and AD using both subcutaneous [40] and intravenous hydrocortisone (fig. 3) [41] infusions. This has paved the way for experimental study designs using this novel concept to address safety, efficacy and clinical outcomes. Øksnes et al. [42] compared the use of CSHI with thrice-daily oral hydrocortisone in their randomized, open-label prospective crossover study conducted in adults with AD in Nor-

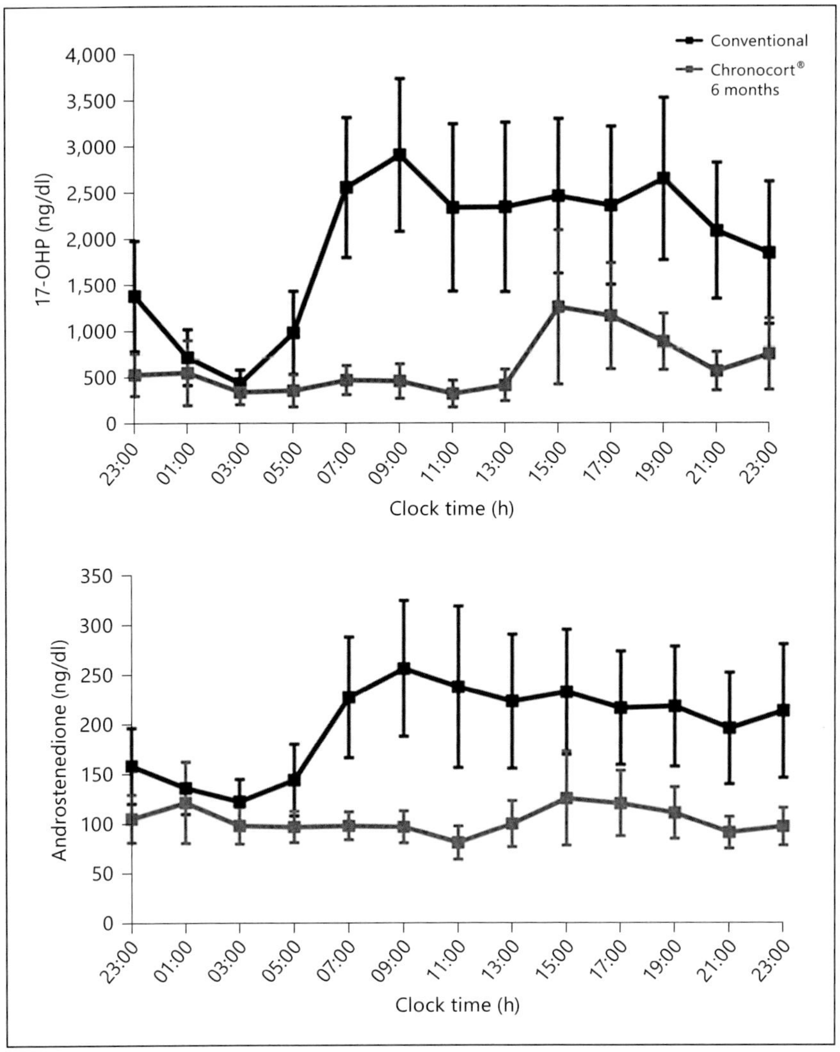


**Fig. 2.** Twenty-four-hour 17-OHP and androstenedione hormone levels on conventional versus Chronocort® therapy. Chronocort® resulted in lower 24-hour, morning (07:00–15:00 h) and afternoon (15:00–23:00 h) androstenedione AUC, and lower 24-hour and morning 17-OHP AUC. Means ± SEM (republished with permission from the Endocrine Society [37]).

way and Sweden. CSHI was able to achieve higher nighttime cortisol AUC (00:00–08:00) which normalized the morning ACTH levels along with achieving morning serum cortisol levels within the reference range. Significant improvements were noted in QOL but bias, given the open-label nature of study, needs to be taken into account. Metabolic improvements may also result from CSHI. By replicating the cortisol rhythm, compared to thrice-daily oral hydrocortisone, the hydrocortisone pump prevented decreasing glucose levels during the night and normalized ACTH levels in patients with AD [43].

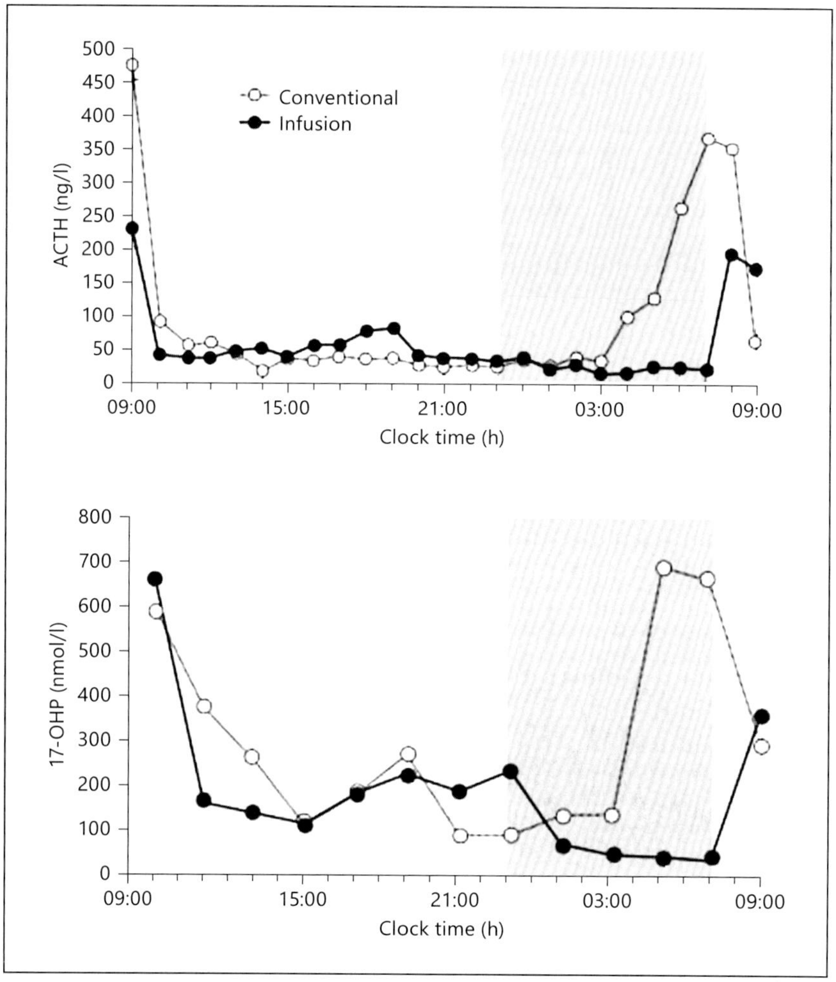


**Fig. 3.** Twenty-four-hour ACTH and 17-OHP levels on conventional oral hydrocortisone versus circadian hydrocortisone intravenous infusion in 2 CAH patients (republished with permission from John Wiley and Sons [41]).

CSHI use in 1 poorly controlled CAH patient has shown dramatic improvements in androgens (17-OHP) [40]. Further studies in additional patients are necessary. Practicality of use is a limitation with this therapy. CSHI is suitable only in willing patients followed regularly but may be useful in patients with gastric side effects from oral treatment or in those with metabolic side effects of glucocorticoid treatment. Furthermore, in states such as puberty, when there is an increase in GH levels leading to an increase in glomerular filtration rate and impairing 11β-hydroxysteroid dehydrogenase type 1 activity, resulting in increased cortisol clearance and decreased tissue cortisol exposure, respectively, it is sometimes impossible to compensate by increasing the frequency of oral dosing, and, in this situation, hydrocortisone infusions could be a suitable alternative [40].

## Conclusions and Future Directions

Newer hydrocortisone formulations and delivery options have brought us closer to replacing cortisol in a more physiological manner. As current health care delivery systems focus more and more towards a personalized medicine model, promising results from these recent advancements are definitely a step forward in the right direction. Further long-term, well-designed clinical trials to assess the effects of physiological cortisol replacement on patient- and disease-related outcomes in both adults and children are necessary.

## Disclosure Statement

No disclosures.

## References


1 Stratmann M, Schibler U: Properties, entrainment, and physiological functions of mammalian peripheral oscillators. J Biol Rhythms 2006;21:494–506.

2 Debono M, Ghobadi C, Rostami-Hodjegan A, et al: Modified-release hydrocortisone to provide circadian cortisol profiles. J Clin Endocrinol Metab 2009; 94:1548–1554.

3 Pezuk P, Mohawk JA, Wang LA, Menaker M: Glucocorticoids as entraining signals for peripheral circadian oscillators. Endocrinology 2012;153:4775–4783.

4 So AY, Bernal TU, Pillsbury ML, et al: Glucocorticoid regulation of the circadian clock modulates glucose homeostasis. Proc Natl Acad Sci U S A 2009; 106:17582–17587.

5 Bostock S, Steptoe A: Influences of early shift work on the diurnal cortisol rhythm, mood and sleep: within-subject variation in male airline pilots. Psychoneuroendocrinology 2013;38:533–541.

6 Desir D, Van Cauter E, Fang VS, et al: Effects of 'jet lag' on hormonal patterns. I. Procedures, variations in total plasma proteins, and disruption of adrenocorticotropin-cortisol periodicity. J Clin Endocrinol Metab 1981;52:628–641.

7 Scheer FA, Hilton MF, Mantzoros CS, Shea SA: Adverse metabolic and cardiovascular consequences of circadian misalignment. Proc Natl Acad Sci U S A 2009;106:4453–4458.

8 Bensing S, Brandt L, Tabaroj F, et al: Increased death risk and altered cancer incidence pattern in patients with isolated or combined autoimmune primary adrenocortical insufficiency. Clin Endocrinol (Oxf) 2008;69:697–704.

9 Filipsson H, Monson JP, Koltowska-Haggstrom M, et al: The impact of glucocorticoid replacement regimens on metabolic outcome and comorbidity in hypopituitary patients. J Clin Endocrinol Metab 2006; 91:3954–3961.

10 Ragnarsson O, Nystrom HF, Johannsson G: Glucocorticoid replacement therapy is independently associated with reduced bone mineral density in women with hypopituitarism. Clin Endocrinol (Oxf) 2012;76:246–252.

11 Hahner S, Loeffler M, Fassnacht M, et al: Impaired subjective health status in 256 patients with adrenal insufficiency on standard therapy based on cross-sectional analysis. J Clin Endocrinol Metab 2007;92: 3912–3922.

12 Lovas K, Husebye ES, Holsten F, Bjorvatn B: Sleep disturbances in patients with Addison's disease. Eur J Endocrinol 2003;148:449–456.

13 Heshmati HM, Riggs BL, Burritt MF, et al: Effects of the circadian variation in serum cortisol on markers of bone turnover and calcium homeostasis in normal postmenopausal women. J Clin Endocrinol Metab 1998;83:751–756.

14 Plat L, Byrne MM, Sturis J, et al: Effects of morning cortisol elevation on insulin secretion and glucose regulation in humans. Am J Physiol 1996;270:E36–E42.

15 Dinneen S, Alzaid A, Miles J, Rizza R: Metabolic effects of the nocturnal rise in cortisol on carbohydrate metabolism in normal humans. J Clin Invest 1993; 92:2283–2290.

16 Langenheim J, Ventz M, Hinz A, Quinkler M: Modified-release prednisone decreases complaints and fatigue compared to standard prednisolone in patients with adrenal insufficiency. Horm Metab Res 2013;45:96–101.
17 Cambiaso P, Schiaffini R, Pontrelli G, et al: Nocturnal hypoglycaemia in ACTH and GH deficient children: role of continuous glucose monitoring. Clin Endocrinol (Oxf) 2013;79:232–237.
18 Zueger T, Kirchner P, Herren C, et al: Glucocorticoid replacement and mortality in patients with nonfunctioning pituitary adenoma. J Clin Endocrinol Metab 2012;97:E1938–E1942.
19 Bleicken B, Hahner S, Loeffler M, et al: Influence of hydrocortisone dosage scheme on health-related quality of life in patients with adrenal insufficiency. Clin Endocrinol (Oxf) 2010;72:297–304.
20 Speiser PW, Azziz R, Baskin LS, et al: Congenital adrenal hyperplasia due to steroid 21-hydroxylase deficiency: an Endocrine Society clinical practice guideline. J Clin Endocrinol Metab 2010;95:4133–4160.
21 Arlt W, Willis DS, Wild SH, et al: Health status of adults with congenital adrenal hyperplasia: a cohort study of 203 patients. J Clin Endocrinol Metab 2010; 95:5110–5121.
22 Finkielstain GP, Kim MS, Sinaii N, et al: Clinical characteristics of a cohort of 244 patients with congenital adrenal hyperplasia. J Clin Endocrinol Metab 2012;97:4429–4438.
23 Han TS, Krone N, Willis DS, et al: Quality of life in adults with congenital adrenal hyperplasia relates to glucocorticoid treatment, adiposity and insulin resistance: United Kingdom Congenital adrenal Hyperplasia Adult Study Executive (CaHASE). Eur J Endocrinol 2013;168:887–893.
24 Merke DP, Poppas DP: Management of adolescents with congenital adrenal hyperplasia. Lancet Diabetes Endocrinol 2013;1:341–352.
25 Charmandari E, Brook CG, Hindmarsh PC: Classic congenital adrenal hyperplasia and puberty. Eur J Endocrinol 2004;151(suppl 3):U77–U82.
26 Debono M, Ross RJ, Newell-Price J: Inadequacies of glucocorticoid replacement and improvements by physiological circadian therapy. Eur J Endocrinol 2009;160:719–729.
27 Simon N, Castinetti F, Ouliac F, et al: Pharmacokinetic evidence for suboptimal treatment of adrenal insufficiency with currently available hydrocortisone tablets. Clin Pharmacokinet 2010;49:455–463.
28 Thomson AH, Devers MC, Wallace AM, et al: Variability in hydrocortisone plasma and saliva pharmacokinetics following intravenous and oral administration to patients with adrenal insufficiency. Clin Endocrinol (Oxf) 2007;66:789–796.
29 Husebye ES, Allolio B, Arlt W, et al: Consensus statement on the diagnosis, treatment and follow-up of patients with primary adrenal insufficiency. J Intern Med 2014;275:104–115.
30 Mah PM, Jenkins RC, Rostami-Hodjegan A, et al: Weight-related dosing, timing and monitoring hydrocortisone replacement therapy in patients with adrenal insufficiency. Clin Endocrinol (Oxf) 2004; 61:367–375.
31 Ekman B, Bachrach-Lindstrom M, Lindstrom T, et al: A randomized, double-blind crossover study comparing two- and four-dose hydrocortisone regimen with regard to quality of life, cortisol and ACTH profiles in patients with primary adrenal insufficiency. Clin Endocrinol (Oxf) 2012;77:18–25.
32 Moeller H: Chronopharmacology of hydrocortisone and 9 alpha-fluorhydrocortisone in the treatment for congenital adrenal hyperplasia. Eur J Pediatr 1985; 144:370–373.
33 Johannsson G, Bergthorsdottir R, Nilsson AG, et al: Improving glucocorticoid replacement therapy using a novel modified-release hydrocortisone tablet: a pharmacokinetic study. Eur J Endocrinol 2009;161: 119–130.
34 Johannsson G, Nilsson AG, Bergthorsdottir R, et al: Improved cortisol exposure-time profile and outcome in patients with adrenal insufficiency: a prospective randomized trial of a novel hydrocortisone dual-release formulation. J Clin Endocrinol Metab 2012;97:473–481.
35 Nilsson AG, Marelli C, Fitts D, et al: Prospective evaluation of long-term safety of dual-release hydrocortisone replacement administered once daily in patients with adrenal insufficiency. Eur J Endocrinol 2014;171:369–377.
36 Verma S, Vanryzin C, Sinaii N, et al: A pharmacokinetic and pharmacodynamic study of delayed- and extended-release hydrocortisone (Chronocort) vs. conventional hydrocortisone (Cortef) in the treatment of congenital adrenal hyperplasia. Clin Endocrinol (Oxf) 2010;72:441–447.
37 Mallappa A, Sinaii N, Kumar P, et al: A phase 2 study of Chronocort, a modified-release formulation of hydrocortisone, in the treatment of adults with classic congenital adrenal hyperplasia. J Clin Endocrinol Metab 2015;100:1137–1145.
38 Whitaker M, Debono M, Huatan H, et al: An oral multiparticulate, modified-release, hydrocortisone replacement therapy that provides physiological cortisol exposure. Clin Endocrinol (Oxf) 2014;80:554–561.
39 Russell GM, Durant C, Ataya A, et al: Subcutaneous pulsatile glucocorticoid replacement therapy. Clin Endocrinol 2014;81:289–293.

40 Hindmarsh PC: The child with difficult to control congenital adrenal hyperplasia: is there a place for continuous subcutaneous hydrocortisone therapy. Clin Endocrinol (Oxf) 2014;81:15–18.
41 Merza Z, Rostami-Hodjegan A, Memmott A, et al: Circadian hydrocortisone infusions in patients with adrenal insufficiency and congenital adrenal hyperplasia. Clin Endocrinol (Oxf) 2006;65:45–50.
42 Øksnes M, Björnsdottir S, Isaksson M, et al: Continuous subcutaneous hydrocortisone infusion versus oral hydrocortisone replacement for treatment of Addison's disease: a randomized clinical trial. J Clin Endocrinol Metab 2014;99:1665–1674.
43 Björnsdottir S, Øksnes M, Isaksson M, et al: Circadian hormone profiles and insulin sensitivity in patients with Addison's disease: a comparison of continuous subcutaneous hydrocortisone infusion with conventional glucocorticoid replacement therapy. Clin Endocrinol (Oxf) 2015;83:28–35.

Dr. Miguel Debono, MD, MRCP, PhD
Academic Unit of Endocrinology, E Floor
The Medical School, University of Sheffield
Beech Hill Road, Sheffield S10 2RX (UK)
E-Mail m.debono@sheffield.ac.uk

Cappa M, Cianfarani S, Ghizzoni L, Loche S, Maghnie M (eds): Advanced Therapies in Pediatric Endocrinology and Diabetology. Endocr Dev. Basel, Karger, 2016, vol 30, pp 54–59 (DOI: 10.1159/000439330)

# Experience with the Histrelin Implant in Pediatric Patients

Erica A. Eugster

Department of Pediatrics, Riley Hospital for Children, Indiana University School of Medicine, Indianapolis, Ind., USA

**Abstract**

The histrelin implant has emerged as a therapeutic option for the treatment of central precocious puberty that has been favorably received by patients and providers. Inserted subcutaneously, the 50-mg implant provides continuous release of the potent gonadotropin-releasing hormone analog (GnRHa) histrelin. Profound suppression of the hypothalamic-pituitary-gonadal (HPG) axis occurs within 1 month of its placement resulting in pubertal arrest, attenuation of skeletal advancement and a progressive increase in predicted adult height. Although marketed for annual use, suppression lasting 2 years from a single implant has been demonstrated. Placing and removing the device is a minor outpatient procedure easily accomplished by a pediatric surgeon using local anesthesia. The major downside to the implant is a ~25% rate of breakage upon removal. Information about the recovery of the HPG axis following histrelin explantation is limited but suggests an average time to menarche comparable with depot GnRHa formulations albeit with wide individual variation.



The histrelin subcutaneous implant was approved for the treatment of central precocious puberty (CPP) in the US in 2007 [1]. The implant, which is constructed of a flexible nonbiodegradable hydrogel, provides continuous release of the drug across microporous walls. The synthetic gonadotropin-releasing hormone analog (GnRHa) histrelin is >200 times more potent than native GnRH and has been commercially available for more than two decades [2]. However, because it previously required daily subcutaneous administration, histrelin became largely obsolete once monthly depot GnRHa preparations were developed [3]. Histrelin reemerged in the therapeutic armamentarium in the form of a yearly implant for the treatment of prostate cancer [4], which paved the way for studies in children with CPP [5]. Although the implants prescribed for these two indications both contain 50 mg of the drug, the device developed for children allows for a more rapid release of histrelin than the one used in adults (65 vs. 41 μg/day). The device is inserted using a trocar, usually by a pediatric surgeon. Although the majority of centers perform the procedure using local anesthesia, conscious sedation and general anesthesia have also been utilized in select cases. Since its approval, the histrelin implant has rapidly increased in popularity in the United States and is now well established as a highly efficacious treatment [6]. However, data regarding long-term follow-up of children treated with this modality are not yet available [7].

## Treatment of Central Precocious Puberty

The first report of the use of the histrelin implant in children involved a pilot study of 11 girls with CPP, all of whom had previously been treated with a depot GnRHa preparation [8]. Serial GnRH stimulation tests demonstrated lower gonadotropin levels after insertion of the implant than on the depot GnRHa with continued hypothalamic-pituitary-gonadal (HPG) axis suppression throughout the treatment course. No difference in biochemical or clinical parameters was seen in patients in whom the implant was replaced at 9 months (n = 5) versus at 15 months (n = 6). Quality of life questionnaires found significantly lower rates of discomfort/pain and less disruption of activities during treatment with the implant than with depot GnRHa intramuscular injections. Following this small trial, an open-label phase III multicenter study was undertaken that involved 36 children (3 boys) from 9 different centers, 20 of whom were naïve to GnRHa therapy. In both naïve and previously treated patients, peak stimulated luteinizing hormone (LH) significantly decreased within 1 month, and estradiol decreased to prepubertal levels in naïve girls. Linear growth velocity and the ratio of bone age to chronological age also declined during the initial year of treatment, while percentiles of body mass index remained stable [9]. Two-year results in 31 children from this same trial demonstrated a further decline in peak stimulated LH at 24 compared with 12 months as well as an increase in predicted adult height (PAH) of 5.1 cm [10]. Final results from the extension phase of this multicenter study are now available. In children completing 6 years of treatment with sequential histrelin implants, pubertal suppression was maintained, bone/chronological age ratio progressively decreased and PAH increased. The greatest gain was observed in treatment-naïve children, who experienced an increase of 10.5 cm in PAH at the end of the trial. No adverse effect on growth velocity or HPG axis recovery was seen, and the implant was well tolerated overall [11].

An important advance in the use of the histrelin implant for CPP was the demonstration that a single implant is effective for 2 years. This was based on the recognition that if 65 μg of drug is released each day, a 50-mg implant should theoretically contain ample histrelin to maintain HPG suppression for 769 days, or exactly 2 years. That this is indeed the case was established by a study involving 33 children with CPP in whom a single implant was left in situ for 2 years. Peak stimulated LH at 12 and 24 months was equivalent, whereas radiographic and clinical indices of puberty progressively improved [12]. Use of a single implant for 2 years has the distinct advantage of significantly decreasing costs and numbers of surgical procedures, and thus has become standard practice at many institutions [pers. commun.].

## Surgical and Anesthetic Considerations

A systematic review of a surgeon's experience with histrelin implant procedures largely corroborates what has been reported in clinical trials. Of 114 cases, ~50% were implantations, 25% were explantations, and 25% were removals followed by insertion of a new implant. The vast majority (95%) of procedures were performed using local anesthesia, with general anesthesia employed primarily in neurologically impaired children [13]. Inhaled nitrous oxide was utilized to augment local anesthesia in this series, although distraction using 'child life' personnel is a less invasive and highly successful alternative approach [pers. experience]. At this author's institution, procedures involving the histrelin implant are also performed primarily by a single pediatric surgeon. Our surgeon reports an average duration of 16.6 min, although with a range of 3–55 min. A longer duration has been noted if the procedure is removal of an implant versus placement (21.6 vs. 10 min, $p < 0.0001$) [unpubl. data].

## Safety

Minor implant site reactions are the most common adverse event reported in patients treated with the histrelin implant and occur in ~50% of patients. These are self-limited and resolve spontaneously. The most troubling safety concern associated with the implant has been a relatively high rate of implant breakage and or difficulty with localization. These issues are limited to the explantation procedure and appear to be due to encapsulation of the device or the presence of scar tissue. Anecdotally, implants appear to become quite desiccated and brittle in some children [pers. commun.] although individual patient characteristics that predict these problems have not been identified. Depending on the study, the rate of implant breakage ranges from 22 to 39% and is higher when left in place for 2 years. Other rarely reported complications have included infection, implant extrusion and keloid scar formation [5]. When intact or partial implants are difficult to localize due to fracture or migration from the insertion site, ultrasonography has been reported to be an effective modality to aid in the retrieval process [14].

## Monitoring

The optimal strategy for monitoring therapy in children being treated for CPP has not been identified, and clinical practice varies significantly among providers. While there is general consensus regarding the importance of following clinical and auxological parameters such as Tanner staging, growth velocity and skeletal maturation, the role of routine hormonal measurements is controversial [15]. The shortage of synthetic GnRH in the US has led to alternative approaches for both the diagnosis and monitoring of children with CPP. One of these has been the use of random ultrasensitive LH values, which have been shown to correlate well with peak stimulated LH at the time of initial presentation [16]. Given the inherent appeal of a simpler and less invasive option than a full stimulation test, it is perhaps not surprising that random LH concentrations have also been applied to the monitoring arena. Interestingly, however, random LH has been shown to often remain in a pubertal range even in patients who have a fully suppressed HPG axis by every other criterion [17]. This phenomenon has been demonstrated during treatment with the histrelin implant as well as with depot leuprolide injections [18]. Thus, random ultrasensitive LH measurements do not have a place in the monitoring of children undergoing treatment for CPP. Whether any biochemical assessment aids in the management of children with CPP who are responding as expected to GnRHa treatment remains to be seen.

## Recovery of the Hypothalamic-Pituitary-Gonadal Axis

Limited information is available thus far regarding the recovery of the HPG axis following treatment with the histrelin implant. In one study, time from explantation to menarche was determined in 11 girls, all but 2 of whom were previously treated with depot GnRHa injections, and was compared to 23 girls treated only with depot GnRHa. The average time to menarche was significantly shorter in the histrelin group compared with the injection group (9.3 vs. 16 months, $p = 0.02$) [19]. In contrast, a larger study involving 30 girls with CPP found an average interval from implant removal to menarche of 12.75 months, albeit with significant individual variation. Of all variables analyzed, only older age at explantation correlated with a shorter duration to menarche. All boys experienced an increase in testicular volume within 1 year of cessation of histrelin implant therapy [20]. While a peak stimulated LH >4 mIU/ml is clearly indicative of reactivation of the reproductive system, there is evidence that free α subunit might represent the earliest detectable biochemical change following removal of the histrelin implant. Rising paradoxically during treatment, free α-subunit concentrations have been shown to fall rapidly upon removal of the implant, preceding changes in sex steroids and gonadotropins by several weeks [21]. An additional advantage of this test is the ability to use it to determine whether an implant has been completely removed in cases where there has been breakage or difficulty with localization.

## Future Directions

Many questions remain regarding the histrelin implant. In the short term, the absolute upper limit of efficacy of the device has not been established. While the implant clearly lasts for at least 2 years, continued suppression of the HPG axis beyond this is theoretically possible. A second logical question is whether the device could be altered in some way as to make breakage and/or problems with localization less of a problem. Additionally, although there are significant data regarding long-term follow-up of children treated with depot GnRHa [22], essentially no such information exists for the histrelin implant. Outcomes of interest include, but are not limited to, reproductive function, bone mineral density and body mass index. Whether CPP is associated with significant psychological problems and, if so, whether treatment with the histrelin implant or other GnRHa formulations alleviates these issues are also areas in which a deficit of knowledge exists [23]. Finally, it will be interesting to observe to what extent the histrelin implant is embraced as a therapeutic modality for CPP in Europe and other parts of the world as compared to its popularity in the US.

## Conclusions

Although the histrelin implant is a relative newcomer to the cadre of GnRHa preparations for the treatment of CPP, studies conducted thus far have consistently demonstrated excellent efficacy of the device in terms of pubertal suppression, including when a single implant is left in place for 2 years. While generally well tolerated, implant breakage and or problems with localization occur in approximately one fourth of patients at the time of removal. Large-scale prospective studies will provide additional important information regarding efficacy, safety and long-term outcomes of children being treated with the histrelin implant for CPP.

## References


1 Nebesio TD, Eugster EA: The histrelin subdermal implant – new treatment for children with central precocious puberty. Rev Endocrinol 2007, pp 39–41.

2 Barradell LB, McTavish D: Histrelin. A review of its pharmacological properties and therapeutic role in central precocious puberty. Drugs 1993;45:570–588.

3 Brito VN, Latronico AC, Arnhold IJ, Mendonça BB: Update on the etiology, diagnosis and therapeutic management of sexual precocity. Arq Bras Endocrinol Metabol 2008;52:18–31.

4 Djavan B, Schlegel P, Salomon G, Eckersberger E, Sadri H, Graefen M: Analysis of testosterone suppression in men receiving histrelin, a novel GnRH agonist for the treatment of prostate cancer. Can J Urol 2010;17:5265–5271.

5 Nebesio TD, Eugster EA: Current concepts in normal and abnormal puberty. Curr Probl Pediatr Adolesc Health Care 2007;37:50–72.

6 Lewis KA, Eugster EA: Experience with the once-yearly histrelin (GnRHa) subcutaneous implant in the treatment of central precocious puberty. Drug Des Devel Ther 2009;3:1–5.

7 Fuqua JS: Treatment and outcomes of precocious puberty: an update. J Clin Endocrinol Metab 2013; 98:2198–2207.
8 Hirsch HJ, Gillis D, Strich D, Chertin B, Farkas A, Lindenberg T, Gelber H, Spitz IM: The histrelin implant: a novel treatment for central precocious puberty. Pediatrics 2005;116:e798–e802.
9 Eugster EA, Clarke W, Kletter GB, Lee PA, Neely EK, Reiter EO, Saenger P, Shulman D, Silverman L, Flood L, Gray W, Tierney D: Efficacy and safety of histrelin subdermal implant in children with central precocious puberty: a multicenter trial. J Clin Endocrinol Metab 2007;92:1697–1704.
10 Rahhal S, Clarke WL, Kletter GB, Lee PA, Neely EK, Reiter EO, Saenger P, Shulman D, Silverman L, Eugster EA: Results of a second year of therapy with the 12-month histrelin implant for the treatment of central precocious puberty. Int J Pediatr Endocrinol 2009;2009:812517.
11 Silverman LA, Neely EK, Kletter GB, Lewis K, Chitra S, Terleckyj O, Eugster EA: Long-term continuous suppression with once-yearly histrelin subcutaneous implants for the treatment of central precocious puberty: a final report of a phase 3 multicenter trial. J Clin Endocrinol Metab 2015;100:2354–2363.
12 Lewis KA, Goldyn AK, West KW, Eugster EA: A single histrelin implant is effective for 2 years for treatment of central precocious puberty. J Pediatr 2013; 163:1214–1216.
13 Davis JS, Alkhoury F, Burnweit C: Surgical and anesthetic considerations in histrelin capsule implantation for the treatment of precocious puberty. J Pediatr Surg 2014;49:807–810.
14 Monroe BJ, Fallon SC, Brandt ML: Intraoperative sonographic localization of a fractured Supprelin implant in a pediatric patient: a case report. J Pediatr Endocrinol Metab 2012;25:167–169.
15 Carel JC, Eugster EA, Rogol A, Ghizzoni L, Palmert MR; ESPE-LWPES GnRH Analogs Consensus Conference Group, Antoniazzi F, Berenbaum S, Bourguignon JP, Chrousos GP, Coste J, Deal S, de Vries L, Foster C, Heger S, Holland J, Jahnukainen K, Juul A, Kaplowitz P, Lahlou N, Lee MM, Lee P, Merke DP, Neely EK, Oostdijk W, Phillip M, Rosenfield RL, Shulman D, Styne D, Tauber M, Wit JM: Consensus statement on the use of gonadotropin-releasing hormone analogs in children. Pediatrics 2009;123:e752–e762.
16 Houk CP, Kunselman AR, Lee PA: Adequacy of a single unstimulated luteinizing hormone level to diagnose central precocious puberty in girls. Pediatrics 2009;123:e1059–e1063.
17 Lewis KA, Eugster EA: Random luteinizing hormone often remains pubertal in children treated with the histrelin implant for central precocious puberty. J Pediatr 2013;162:562–565.
18 Neely EK, Lee PA, Bloch CA, Larsen L, Yang D, Mattia-Goldberg C, Chwalisz K: Leuprolide acetate 1-month depot for central precocious puberty: hormonal suppression and recovery. Int J Pediatr Endocrinol 2010;2010:398639.
19 Gillis D, Karavani G, Hirsch HJ, Strich D: Time to menarche and final height after histrelin implant treatment for central precocious puberty. J Pediatr 2013;163:532–536.
20 Fisher MM, Lemay D, Eugster EA: Resumption of puberty in girls and boys following removal of the histrelin implant. J Pediatr 2014;164:912–916.
21 Hirsch HJ, Lahlou N, Gillis D, Strich D, Rosenberg-Hagen B, Chertin B, Farkas A, Hartman H, Spitz IM: Free alpha-subunit is the most sensitive marker of gonadotropin recovery after treatment of central precocious puberty with the histrelin implant. J Clin Endocrinol Metab 2010;95:2841–2844.
22 Thornton P, Silverman LA, Geffner ME, Neely EK, Gould E, Danoff TM: Review of outcomes after cessation of gonadotropin-releasing hormone agonist treatment of girls with precocious puberty. Pediatr Endocrinol Rev 2014;11:306–317.
23 Schoelwer M, Donohue K, Bryk K, Didrick P, Berenbaum S, Eugster EA: Psychological assessment of mothers and their daughters at the time of diagnosis of precocious puberty. Int J Pediatr Endocrinol 2015; 2015:5.

Erica A. Eugster, MD
Pediatric Endocrinology #5960
Department of Pediatrics
Riley Hospital for Children
Indiana University School of Medicine
705 Riley Hospital Drive, Indianapolis, IN 46202 (USA)
E-Mail eeugster@iu.edu

Cappa M, Cianfarani S, Ghizzoni L, Loche S, Maghnie M (eds): Advanced Therapies in Pediatric Endocrinology and Diabetology. Endocr Dev. Basel, Karger, 2016, vol 30, pp 60–78 (DOI: 10.1159/000439332)

# Different Medications for Hypogonadotropic Hypogonadism

Giulia Rastrelli · Linda Vignozzi · Mario Maggi

Sexual Medicine and Andrology Unit, Department of Experimental and Clinical Biomedical Sciences Mario Serio, University of Florence, Florence, Italy

**Abstract**

Delayed puberty (DP) in boys is the lack of sexual maturation at a chronological age of 14 years. Several conditions induce DP and they can be classified into reversible and irreversible causes. The most common cause of DP is constitutional delay of puberty (CDP; 63%), followed by DPs due to functional hypogonadotropic hypogonadism (HH; 20%), congenital isolated HH (9%) and hypergonadotropic hypogonadism (7%). A correct diagnosis, although often difficult, is pivotal for choosing the most adequate therapy. In CDP boys, expectant management can be an option. However, patient's psychological distress can be attenuated by short-term low-dose testosterone therapy, which can induce male secondary sexual characteristics. When therapy is discontinued in CDP, pubertal development continues similarly to normal boys. Long-term testosterone therapy is the only option in boys with DP due to hypergonadotropic hypogonadism, whereas in subjects with HH, besides long-term testosterone, also gonadotropins and gonadotropin-releasing hormone (GnRH) can be used. Gonadotropins and GnRH, besides inducing secondary sexual characteristics, can also induce testicular maturation and spermatogenesis. Other molecules, such as kisspeptin and neurokinin B agonists, are now under evaluation as new therapeutic options for treating DP.



Puberty is the physiological process of physical and psychological modifications that leads from childhood to adulthood. During this period, sexual characteristics and reproductive capability are acquired. In addition, several psychological modifications, known as adolescence, give people problem-solving and -coping abilities, as well as self-identity and independence from the nuclear family.

Puberty is due to a reactivation of pulsatile secretion of gonadotropin-releasing hormone (GnRH) from the hypothalamus which, in turn, causes an episodic secretion of luteinizing hormone (LH) and follicle-stimulating hormone (FSH) from the pituitary, which stimulate the testicular production of testosterone and spermatogenesis.

Following an intense activity during fetal life and early childhood, the hypothalamic-pituitary-testis axis remains quiescent until puberty, when pulsatile GnRH-gonadotropin secretion restarts. The mechanisms that contribute to the 're-awakening' of the hypothalamic-pituitary-testis axis are still largely unknown. It has been hypothesized that an interplay between neuronal, endocrine and nutritional factors acts on the hypothalamus, giving both positive and negative stimuli for GnRH secretion.

## Physiology of Puberty

GnRH neurons are a small number of cells that, at the beginning of embryonic life, originate in the nasal placode and, during development, migrate first into the nasal compartment, then through the cribriform plate and, finally, through the basal forebrain, before they take their positions in the arcuate nucleus of the hypothalamus. The correct establishment and ending of this GnRH neuron 'journey' is extremely important for the onset of puberty and maintenance of reproduction. Failure of GnRH neurons to migrate leads to a clinical condition defined as congenital isolated hypogonadotropic hypogonadism (ciHH) that, if associated with anosmia, is also known as Kallmann's syndrome. Besides reaching the correct position within the hypothalamus, GnRH neurons also have to receive apposition of kisspeptin/neurokinin B (NKB)/dynorphin (KNDy) positive cells, which are considered to be the main GnRH pulse regulators. Loss-of-function mutations in the genes encoding NKB *(NKB)* and its cognate receptor, TAK3R, or the kisspeptin *(KiSS-1)* and its receptor G-protein-coupled receptor 54 *(GPR54*, now called *KiSS-1R)* result in normosmic congenital HH with the absence of pubertal development. A crucial role in puberty and reproduction is played by *KiSS*-1R and its natural ligand, the product of the *KiSS-1* gene, kisspeptin-54. The KiSS-*1*/*KiSS-1R* system was first unraveled by the finding that inactivating mutations in the *KiSS-1R* gene were associated with a lack of puberty onset and HH both in humans and mice. In human GnRH-secreting neuroblasts (FNC-B4), androgens and leptin (a signal of energy abundance) have been demonstrated to stimulate *KiSS-1*/*KiSS-1R* expression [1] and GnRH release [2], whereas estrogens have a negative effect [1], data in agreement with those reported in previous studies on the rat hypothalamus. The interaction between leptin, as a peripheral signal, and kisspeptin, as a central processor which triggers puberty, has also been demonstrated by experimental animal studies of fasting-induced leptin deficiency, in which inhibition of the reproductive axis was associated with a reduced expression of *KiSS-1* mRNA [3]. The central administration of kisspeptin reversed the inhibition of gonadotropin secretion induced by fasting [3]. Interestingly, in FNC-B4 neuroblasts, leptin treatment induced not only a marked increase in mRNA expression of *KiSS-1*/*KiSS-1R* but also of leptin receptor *(LEPR)* and androgen receptor *(AR)*. On the other hand, dihydrotestosterone treatment also had multiple effects on FNC-B4 neuroblasts, including the induction not only of the *KiSS-1/KiSS-1R* system, but also that of *AR* and *LEPR* [1]. Taken together, these data can at least partially explain the physiology of puberty onset as a result of the interplay among multiple genes and peripheral hormones such as leptin, which is an index of an appropriate nutritional status, and sex steroids, in particular adrenal androgens, which are secreted after adrenarche.

### Physical Modifications during Puberty

The first clinical sign of the onset of puberty in males is the enlargement of the testes and, in particular, the achievement of a testis volume of 4 ml indicates the start of the pubertal development process, usually at 12 ± 2 years [4]. Testicular volume, measured by comparing the testes with ellipsoids of known volume (Prader orchidometer; fig. 1a), can be correlated with the stages of puberty. The phases of genital development are classified and described, according to Tanner, into five stages, from G1 (prepubertal stage) to G5 (adult genitalia in size and shape; fig. 1b). Also, pubic hair development is classified using a similar grading (fig. 1b); however, it cannot be considered as a marker of pubertal progression, since pubic hair appearance is under the control of adrenal, more than testicular, androgens. For this reason, appearance of pubic, as well as axillary hair, is a sign of the adrenarche, a process in terms of time, but not mechanistically, linked to pubertal development. The length of the phallus (excluding the foreskin) increases from an average of 6.2 cm in the prepubertal state to 12.4 ± 2.7 cm in the adult. The phallus is more accurately measured stretched than in the flaccid state as there is much interindividual variation in the length of the unstretched penis. In addition, membranous and cartilaginous components of the vocal cords lengthen during puberty from 12–15 to 18 to 23 mm, and the larynx, cricothyroid cartilage and laryngeal muscles enlarge, resulting in a deepening of the voice. Facial hair development usually occurs during pubic hair stage 3 and is first apparent on the upper lip and upper cheek, then on the lower lip and finally on the sides of the chin. Another topical modification occurring during puberty is the increase in growth velocity that starts at the beginning of puberty, peaks at 14 years and allows a boy to increase in height by 28 cm in 3 years, a phenomenon known as 'growth spurt'. At the same time, bone mineral density increases until the peak of bone mass is reached in early adulthood. Body composition changes and both fat and fat-free mass increase so that a 1:1 ratio is maintained in males during and after puberty. Another crucial modification during puberty is the development of the spermatogenetic function. Sertoli cells are the major cell type in the prepubertal and early pubertal seminiferous tubule, but in adults, a predominance of germ cells is observed. During pubertal progression, Sertoli cells differentiate into adult-type Sertoli cells, establishing occlusive junctions, known as the blood-testicular barrier. With pubertal development and rising serum LH levels,

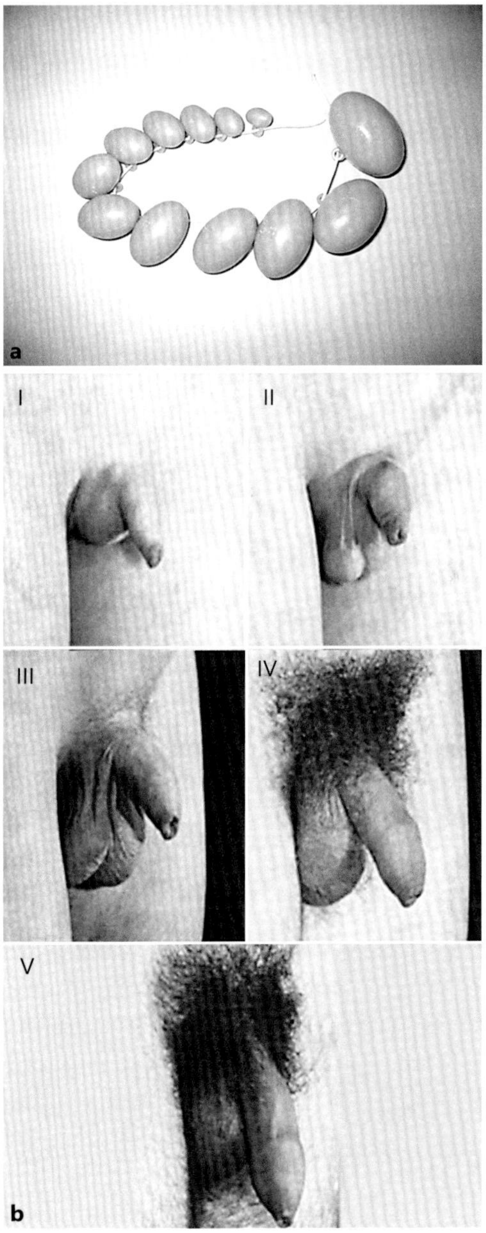


**Fig. 1.** Clinical modifications of male external genitalia according to the Tanner classification. **a** Prader orchidometer. **b** Tanner stages I–V: *pubic hair:* Tanner I = No pubic hair at all; Tanner II = small amount of long, downy hair with slight pigmentation at the base of the penis and scrotum; Tanner III = hair becomes more coarse and curly, and begins to extend laterally; Tanner IV = adult-like hair quality, extending across pubis but sparing medial thighs; Tanner V = hair extends to medial surface of the thighs; *genitals:* Tanner I = prepubertal (testicular volume less than 1.5 ml; small penis of 3 cm or less); Tanner II = testicular volume between 1.6 and 6 ml; skin on scrotum thins, reddens and enlarges; penis length unchanged; Tanner III = testicular volume between 6 and 12 ml; scrotum enlarges further; penis begins to lengthen to about 6 cm; Tanner IV = testicular volume between 12 and 20 ml; scrotum enlarges further and darkens; penis increases in length to 10 cm and in circumference; Tanner V = testicular volume greater than 20 ml; adult scrotum and penis of 15 cm in length.

Leydig cells maturate from undifferentiated mesenchyme-type cells to adult-type Leydig cells. The first histologic evidence of spermatogenesis appears between 11 and 15 years of age, and sperm can be detected in the first morning urine specimen (spermaturia). Spermaturia probably reflects the onset and maturation of spermatogenesis, but normospermia (sperm concentration, morphology and motility) is not present until a bone age of 17 years.

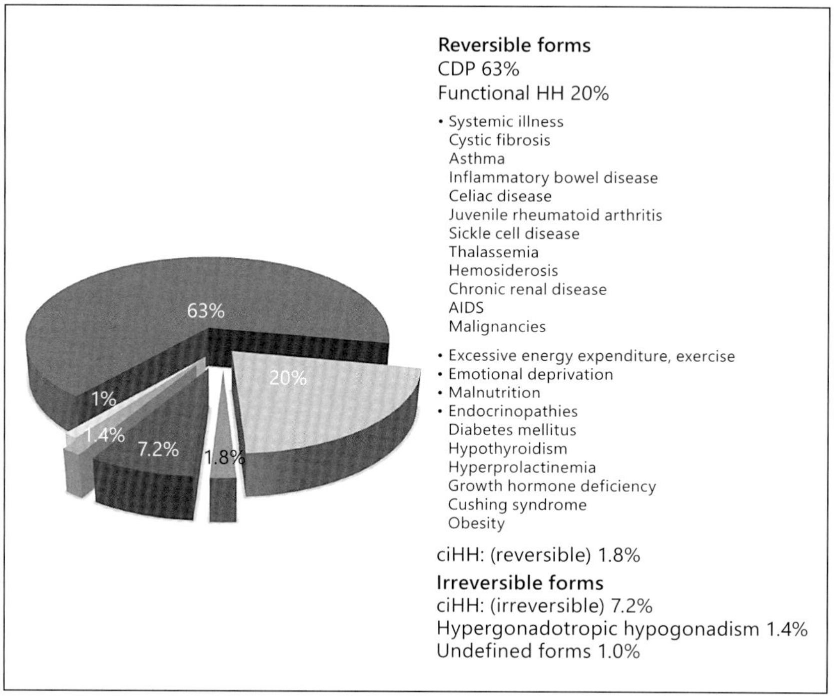


**Fig. 2.** Causes of DP.

## Definition of Delayed Puberty

Delayed puberty (DP) is defined as the lack of development of sexual maturation in boys at a chronological age that is 2.5 standard deviations above the mean age of onset of puberty in a normal population, which corresponds to the absence of signs of puberty by age 14 in the US [4]. DP is twice more common in boys than girls; however, in the US, less than 2% of 14-year-old boys are prepubertal [4].

## Etiology of Delayed Puberty

Several conditions induce DP and they can be classified into reversible and irreversible causes (fig. 2). Among the reversible causes, there is the most common form of DP, the constitutional delay of puberty (CDP; fig. 2). It represents the extreme of the normal timing of puberty onset, since boys with CDP are overall healthy and, by definition, their puberty starts spontaneously by the age of 18 years [5]. CDP is the cause of DP in 63% of boys [6] and, due its benign and self-limiting nature, theoretically it does not need a specific treatment, even though psychological and self-esteem factors, which present secondary to a delay in pubertal development in comparison with peers, should be considered before deciding on expectant observation. CDP is a diagnosis by exclusion, so all the other possible conditions causing DP should be accurately considered. In particular, differential diagnosis with ciHH could be insidious. ciHH is characterized by an impaired GnRH and/or gonadotropic secretion and not accompanied by other hypothalamic and/or pituitary hormone deficiencies; it represents 9% of cases of DP (fig. 2) [6]. As previously mentioned, ciHH is caused by defects in genes involved in the process of the development or migration of GnRH neurons from the nasal placode to the hypothalamus or in the regulation of GnRH secretion or GnRH action, although a genetic diagnosis is reached only in 50% of cases. CDP and HH display similar clinical and biochemical features. An element that could aid in distinguishing these two conditions is that whereas CDP boys usually have a history of delayed growth with short stature but a relatively normal growth rate, ciHH subjects show a normal stature during childhood with a normal growth rate that slows down in the peripubertal period. Furthermore, CDP is also accompanied by a delayed adrenarche, as a consequence of an overall delayed development. Conversely, as a consequence of a hypothalamic-pituitary defect, ciHH does not include a delay in adrenal function, and adrenarche can occur properly. In addition, ciHH boys often show clinical signs of lack of minipuberty, such as cryptorchidism, micropenis or hypospadias, not usually present in CDP boys. Both ciHH and CDP conditions have a considerable rate of familiar cases. It is estimated that at least 80% of the variation in the timing of puberty is due to genetic factors and, accordingly, 50–75% of CDP subjects have a family history of DP [5], although the genes involved are still largely unknown. Concerning ciHH, familiar cases are estimated to be 1 out of 3 [5], and the proportion is likely to be higher, since the list of genes involved in the pathogenesis of the disorder lengthens every day. However, in families of ciHH boys, and in these boys themselves, specific clinical features, such as hypo/anosmia, renal agenesis, cleft lip/palate, iris coloboma and mirror movements, can be found in association or not with hypogonadism. Hence, recognizing one or more of these features in relatives can be of help in diagnosing ciHH instead of CDP. Also, the hormonal pattern is similar in these two conditions, with an overlap of baseline testosterone and gonadotropins. Even if several tests have been proposed for this differential diagnosis, such as testing daily urine excretion of FSH and LH, LH pulsatility assessment, prolactin response to different stimulating agents, GnRH test and human chorionic gonadotropin (hCG) test, none of them has proven to distinguish CDP from ciHH [5]. Recently, Coutant et al. [7] demonstrated that a single baseline measurement of inhibin B can discriminate prepubertal boys with CDP from those with HH, and, in particular, a value lower than 35 pg/ml has a 100% sensitivity and specificity in identifying hypogonadal boys. If confirmed, this method would represent a relatively simple and noninvasive tool for the differential diagnosis of DP. The importance of distinguishing CDP from ciHH lies in the different pathological significance of these conditions and different treatment strategies. In fact, CDP is not a disease at all, whereas ciHH carries the risk of malformations in the subject himself and/or his relatives or possible offspring. Concerning therapy, whereas expectant management or a short-term treatment are possible strategies in CDP, they cannot be undertaken in ciHH boys, whose early diagnosis and treatment is pivotal not only for inducing pubertal development, but also for improving fertility outcomes. However, in contrast with the classical view of ciHH as an irreversible condition, cases of ciHH, with documented genetic defects, have been described as reversed to eugonadism after discontinuation of treatment with either testosterone replacement therapy (TRT), gonadotropins or GnRH [8]. In particular, in a retrospective analysis of more than 300 ciHH subjects, reversal was reported in 20% of cases after the discontinuation of therapy which lasted a mean time of 4.4 years (fig. 2) [9]. As aforementioned, androgens play multiple roles in GnRH neurons, including the induction of KiSS-1R, AR and LEPR expression [1] thus facilitating the activity of the neuronal machinery leading to the 'awakening' and sustained function of GnRH pulse generator. This mechanism can explain the reversal of hypogonadism in ciHH subjects after treatment.

Besides ciHH, deficiency in GnRH and/or gonadotropins is found also in subjects with mutations in genes involved in hypothalamic or pituitary development, such as HESX1, PROP-1, LHX3 and LHX4; however, these mutations cause complex clinical conditions, which are characterized by multiple hypothalamic/pituitary hormone deficiencies as well as cerebral and craniofacial malformations, so DP is a lesser aspect.

Acquired forms of HH are due to chronic diseases, such as systemic illnesses (fig. 2) as well as their medications, endocrine diseases, nutritional or emotional deprivation but also to excessive physical exercise which induce a functional, potentially reversible, GnRH/gonadotropin deficiency that is found as the cause of DP in 20% of cases (fig. 2) [6]. HH can be acquired also due to tumors or infiltrative diseases that damage hypothalamic and pituitary tissue. However, it must be noted that, apart from craniopharyngioma, which usually causes growth and pubertal delay, intracranial diseases often lead to precocious, rather than delayed, puberty. Finally, 7% of DP cases are due to congenital or acquired testicular failure, leading to hypergonadotropic hypogonadism which is an irreversible condition (fig. 2) [6].

## Diagnostic Workup

Since there is a variation in timing of puberty and most causes of DP have a genetic hereditary background, assessment of the family history is important when evaluating boys with DP (fig. 3). In particular, growth patterns, pubertal timing and response to possible therapy for puberty induction in parents and other relatives must be investigated.

Evaluation of growth patterns and development of the patient until the time of first assessment is pivotal for an initial diagnostic assessment (fig. 3). Patients with delayed linear growth, but normal growth velocity, without signs of adrenarche, which is itself delayed, can suggest CDP. On the contrary, subjects whose linear growth has been normal until peripubertal age when a reduction in growth velocity is detected and

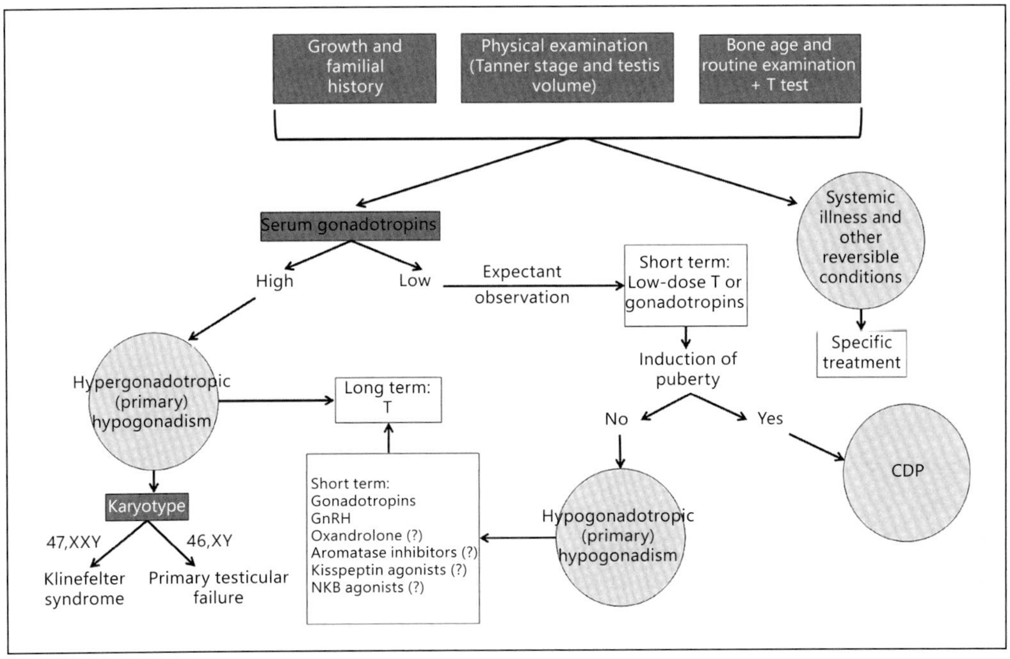


**Fig. 3.** Diagnostic workup in DP. T = Testosterone.

possibly with normal appearance of pubic and axillary hair raise the suspicion of HH. Symptoms and signs of hormone deficiencies (non-isolated HH) or excess (endocrine diseases, such as the Cushing syndrome or hyperprolactinemia) must be assessed. A past history of chronic illnesses, as well as current or previous therapies, presence of symptoms or signs of unrecognized systemic diseases, and emotional or psychological distress must be carefully evaluated (fig. 3).

Physical examination must include height and weight measurements, which must be plotted on a growth chart, where a patient's measurements are compared with those of subjects of the same age (fig. 3). The target height, calculated as the mid-parental height, should be calculated in order to appropriately evaluate the growth trend of the patient and also the response to therapy. Penis length and testis volume must be measured and categorized according to Tanner staging. Testis volume growth is the first sign of starting of puberty, and, in particular, a volume greater than 4 ml is a predictor of a spontaneous occurrence of puberty. Pubic and axillary hair must be observed as signs of adrenarche.

Bone age, which is assessed by specific radiographs, is useful as a predictor of puberty onset, when bone age is 11–12.5 years; however, a delayed bone age in DP subjects does not help with diagnosis because it is not specific to any etiology (fig. 3).

Laboratory tests must include routine analysis for the assessment of markers of systemic diseases and/or inflammation, as well as specific evaluations required on the basis of particular symptoms and signs (fig. 3). Testosterone levels are important to evaluate, since values higher than 1 nmol/l indicate that the puberty process has already started and values higher than 0.7 nmol/l predict puberty onset within 12 months in 77% of cases and within 15 months in 100% of cases. Baseline gonadotropin assessment is pivotal because high levels indicate primary testis failure, an irreversible cause of DP. Diagnosis of hypergonadotropic hypogonadism needs further assessments, first of all karyotyping for Klinefelter's syndrome that, when a patient does not report a history of pelvic trauma, inguinal surgery, chemo- or pelvic radiotherapy, is the most likely diagnosis. In the case of a normal karyotype, rarer causes of primary failure, such as defects of steroidogenesis or autoimmunity, must be considered. Low to normal gonadotropins in prepubertal boys do not add much in differentiating a diagnosis, because they are typical of several causes of DP. Pituitary function should be assessed in specific cases, when symptoms and signs of hormone deficiency or excess are found. Also, magnetic resonance imaging is not routinely required and should be reserved to specific cases, when hormone excess or multiple deficiencies or neurological symptoms, such as headache or visual field defects, are detected. As already mentioned, several attempts to validate laboratory tests for differential diagnosis between CDP and ciHH have been done without definitive success. Quite recently, promising results have been reported for baseline measurement of inhibin B, even though this test is still not routinely used at all. At present, the differential diagnosis is an a posteriori evaluation based on natural history (i.e. expectant management with spontaneous puberty within 18 years or sustained acquisition of hypothalamic-pituitary function after a short-term androgen therapy).

## Therapy

When discussing therapy of DP, treatment of transient or permanent hypogonadism is essentially described [see ref. 10 for review]. In fact, except for hypothalamic-pituitary-testis axis failure due to systemic illnesses, endocrine diseases, malnutrition, emotional deprivation or excessive physical exercise, which can be reversed by the adequate correction of the causal condition, DP treatment relies on the substitution of gonadal function (table 1).

For hypergonadotropic hypogonadism, the only possible therapeutic option is TRT.

In virtue of the self-limiting nature of CDP, expectant management, including correct information of the patient and parents, reassurance and periodical observation, is one therapeutic option. In these boys, puberty starts spontaneously just a few years later than in their peers and follows all the normal steps, leading to a normal, although late, achievement of maturity. Final height spontaneously achieved is that expected based on parental height, although it has been reported that boys whose linear growth decreases in the years before the expected pubertal age will ultimately reach a height significantly lower than the target [5]. However, expectant management has some

**Table 1.** Possible therapies in DP

| Compound | Trade name | Initial dosage | Advantages | Disadvantages | Licensed for DP |
|---|---|---|---|---|---|
| *Testosterone (T)* | | | | | |
| Injectable | | | | | |
| T enanthate | Testoviron Depot®<br>Delatestryl®<br>Testo-Enant® | 50 mg i.m. monthly | Injections every month<br>Cheap<br>Wide experience | Wide T plasma level fluctuations<br>Erythrocytosis | Yes |
| T cypionate | Depo-Testosterone Inj® | | | | |
| T propionate | Testovis® | | | | |
| Oral | | | | | |
| T undecanoate | Andriol®<br>Andriol Testocaps® | 20–40 mg daily | Easy to take<br>Nontoxic<br>Wide experience | Daily administration<br>Unpredictable absorption<br>Wide T plasma level fluctuation | No |
| Transdermal | | | | | |
| Patches | *Not scrotal:*<br>Androderm®<br>Andropatch®<br>Testopatch®<br>Virormone®<br>*Scrotal*<br>Testoderm® | 2.5–5 mg for 12 h daily | Easy to take | Itching and contact dermatitis (~50%)<br>Expensive<br>Low experience in DP | No |
| Gel 1% | AndroGel®<br>Testogel®<br>Testim®<br>Fortigel® | 1.5 mg daily | Easy to take | Expensive<br>Low experience in DP | No |
| Gel 2% | Testostop®<br>Tostrex®<br>Axiron® | | | | |
| Pellet | Testopel®<br>Testolmplant® | 8–10 mg/kg every 4–7 months | Long acting | Invasive and inconvenient to apply<br>Low experience in DP | No |
| *Oxandrolone* | Anavar® | 2.5 mg daily | Easy to take | Risk of hepatotoxicity | No |
| *Letrozole (combined with T)* | Calantha®<br>Femara®<br>Letrix®<br>Zoltron® | 2.5 mg daily | Increase of predicted final adult height | Risk of bone demineralization and delayed maturation | No |
| *Gonadotropins* | *hCG or LH:*<br>Novarel®<br>Chorex®<br>Gonic®<br>Choron®<br>Chorigon®<br>Pregnyl®<br>Gonasi®<br>Profasi®<br>Ovidrel®<br>Ovitrelle® | 1,000 IU twice-thrice weekly | Induction of testicular maturation<br>Induction of spermatogenesis<br>Reduction of time to fertility achievement after TRT | Inconvenient to administer<br>Expensive | Yes |
| | *hMG or FSH*<br>Meropur®<br>Pergoveris®<br>Puregon®<br>Gonal F® | 75 IU thrice weekly | | | No |
| *GnRH* | Factrel®<br>Lutrepulse® | 25 ng/kg every 90–120 min | Induction of testicular maturation<br>Induction of spermatogenesis<br>Reduction of time to fertility achievement after TRT | Inconvenient to administer | Yes |

limitations. Firstly, it is applied without the certainty of the diagnosis that, by definition, is made a posteriori. Furthermore, the growth and sexual and psychological delay in comparison with peers can lead to important distress and is a risk factor for being the victim of bullying. Instead of expectant management, androgen therapy can be offered.

### *Testosterone*

Testosterone preparations can be used in HH and CDP, and they are the only possibility in hypergonadotropic hypogonadism. Irrespective of the nature of the hypogonadism, testosterone therapy should be started at the age of 14 years with 25% of an adult dosage that must be gradually increased until the adult dose is reached over 3–4 years [4]. Several preparations of testosterone are available (table 1) [see ref. 11 for review]. Injectable preparations are those with the widest clinical experience. In particular, testosterone enanthate is started at 50 mg i.m. every 4 weeks and gradually escalated every 6 months to 100–150 mg monthly until achieving maturity, usually in 3–4 years, when the adult protocol (250 mg every 2–3 weeks) is indicated. When suspecting CDP, a short-term testosterone therapy can be attempted for 3 months. After this period, if pubertal development continues to go on, a diagnosis of CDP can be confirmed; if pubertal modifications stop or regress, a second 3-month course of testosterone therapy is indicated, and a lack of spontaneous progression of puberty after the second course of therapy suggests a diagnosis of HH.

Most studies on the use of testosterone in DP are observational, and few randomized clinical trials (RCTs), including small numbers of patients, are available. However, there is a general agreement on the effectiveness of injectable testosterone in inducing an increase in growth rate without negatively affecting the final adult height. Furthermore, injectable testosterone preparations have a satisfactory safety profile. Priapism is an adverse effect, more frequently reported in subjects starting treatment with an initial dose of 100 mg monthly. Since alkylated esters of testosterone are no longer recommended, liver damage is not a concern, and monitoring of hepatic function is not required anymore.

As an alternative to injectable preparations, oral testosterone undecanoate can be considered (table 1). Testosterone undecanoate has the advantage of not being as cumbersome as injections are and, for this reason, it could be useful in young boys. However, it requires daily administration and, more importantly, its absorption is unpredictable and highly dependent on the fat content of meals. In fact, wide plasma level fluctuations are typical of this preparation. Few studies have evaluated testosterone undecanoate in adolescent boys, and the dosage to be used has not been standardized. An initial dose of 20 mg has been used to mimic the rise in testosterone in early puberty [12], and 40 mg has been found to be able to produce testosterone levels in mid-late puberty [13], whereas the usual dosage for adults is 80–160 mg daily.

However, an RCT, involving 16 prepubertal boys aged 11–14 years with constitutional delay of growth, demonstrated that oral testosterone undecanoate, compared to placebo, is able to increase growth rate, but not to induce or maintain the hormonal modifications typical of pubertal development [12]. On the contrary, administration of 40 mg daily in 4 DP boys, aged 12.7–17.1 years, has been reported as effective in initiating puberty [13]. Furthermore, oral testosterone undecanoate 40 mg daily has been compared with Sustanon, an injectable preparation that is a mixture of testosterone propionate, phenylpropionate and isocaproate, in an RCT involving 12 boys with DP with a mean age of 14.3 years. In this study, testosterone undecanoate did not show any difference from injectable testosterone in promoting growth rate and bone mineralization [14]. Oral testosterone undecanoate has wide clinical use, so it can be considered safe for treating adolescent boys with DP; however, it must be stressed that testosterone undecanoate is not licensed for oral use in adolescents with DP.

Transdermal testosterone (gel or patch) is another possible solution (table 1). Patches can be applied to scrotal or nonscrotal skin, and they deliver testosterone into the systemic circulation, thus mimicking circadian rhythms. They are characterized by a limited compliance because adverse skin reactions in the application zone are frequently reported. Only few studies have been conducted using patches in boys. In an open label study conducted in a small sample of boys with thalassemia major, Androderm patch 2.5 mg overnight induced physiologic testosterone levels, with a decrease in sex hormone binding globulin and an increase in growth, virilization and bone mineralization [15]. In a more recent study [16], 8 patients with DP or a history of growth delay, aged 12.4–14.9 years, were randomly assigned to receive Virormone patch 5 mg for 8 or 12 h nightly. This treatment was shown to be able to raise salivary testosterone levels and to stimulate leg growth and bone turnover, without differences between groups. Gels are relatively new formulations introduced in the US in 2000. When applied to the skin, the hydroalcoholic gel is absorbed into the stratum corneum, which forms a reservoir and acts as a rate-controlling membrane. Recommended adult dosage is 5 g/day, which provides a delivery of 5 mg/day. Testosterone gels are colorless, hydroalcoholic gels, formulated with testosterone concentrations of 1 or 2% that provide continuous delivery of testosterone for 24 h after a single-day application. In adult hypogonadal men, they were efficient in achieving testosterone levels in the normal adult range, without fluctuations during the day. They have shown a highly satisfactory safety profile and they are well tolerated by patients, with skin rash as the most frequent concern reported, although less frequent than with patches. These characteristics make testosterone gels appealing also for DP therapy. However, only one study evaluated their use in adolescence [17]. In the Rogol multicenter, open-label study, testosterone gel 1% was administered to 29 adolescents (12–17 years) with primary hypogonadism due to the Klinefelter syndrome or anorchia. Initial dose was 0.5 mg daily, titrated up to 5 mg on the investigator's clinical judgment. In this study, testosterone gel was able to increase serum testosterone levels 2–10 times compared with the baseline values, without causing any serious adverse event, with cough, acne and headache as the most reported complains. Neither testosterone patches nor testosterone gels are licensed for use in adolescents with DP.

TRT can also be performed with subcutaneous pellets, which are made from pure crystals of testosterone, which represent the most long-lasting option (table 1). They are implanted subcutaneously and held with a retention suture; the erosion at their surface leads to systemic absorption. Standard adult dosage is four 200-mg pellets that last 4–7 months providing stable testosterone level concentrations. The use of pellets for treating DP is documented only by one observational study [18] involving 16 patients aged 13.9–17.5 years previously treated by different preparations of testosterone. Testosterone pellets were implanted subcutaneously at a dose of 8–10 mg/kg for 18 months after at least 2 weeks of washout from previous medications. In this study, treatment appropriately maintained the increase in growth rate induced by previous medications. Furthermore, penile growth continued without modifications in testis size. Subjects reported physical and emotional well-being, few adverse events, such as minor infection or fibrosis at the site of pellet insertion, and all of the boys declared to prefer this testosterone preparation to the previous ones used. However, no further study was conducted on this preparation, which had the disadvantage of being invasive and inconvenient to apply. In addition, it must be noted that it is available only in the United States, United Kingdom and Australia, and not licensed for use in adolescents.

### *Other Androgens*

Oxandrolone is a synthetic anabolic steroid and it is a 17α-alkylated derivative of testosterone (2-oxa-17α-hydroxy-methyl-5α-androstan-3-one). Oxandrolone can be considered a selective androgen receptor modulator, since it acts as an androgen without apparent estrogenic effect. For this reason, it is particularly useful in DP, because it can induce growth without the risk of too rapid skeletal maturation (table 1). When given orally, it is well absorbed and reaches the peak of blood concentration after 1 h; then, it is eliminated with a half-life of 9.4 h. The alkylation in the 17α position prevents rapid breakdown in the liver, even though it is burdened by the risk of hepatotoxicity, so that its use is no longer recommended. However, a short course with a low dose of oxandrolone is sometimes used as an alternative to intramuscular testosterone. Its efficacy in the treatment of DP has been evaluated in a small number of RCTs that tested the administration of oxandrolone 2.5 mg daily for 3–6 months given at bedtime in comparison with placebo or injectable testosterone. In these studies, oxandrolone demonstrated an increase in growth velocity and pubertal development that was significantly higher than placebo and not significantly different from testosterone. Since oxandrolone transiently blunts gonadotropin secretion [19], testis volume in boys treated with oxandrolone was not different from the arm receiving placebo or testosterone [20], although other reports describe an increase in testis volume [21, 22].

### *Aromatase Inhibitors*

The use of aromatase inhibitors, in association with testosterone, in boys with DP has been evaluated with the rationale of delaying fusion of epiphyses of the long bones, thus allowing these boys to potentially increase their final adult height (table 1). Most of the studies on this topic have been produced by a single research group which assessed the effects of letrozole 2.5 mg orally in association with testosterone enanthate as compared with testosterone enanthate plus placebo. The authors found that, in boys with DP, the use of letrozole is associated with an increase in predicted adult height with a delay in bone maturation that was not observed in the testosterone-placebo group [23]. The major concern in the use of aromatase inhibitors during adolescence is the deficit in bone mass accretion. In boys treated with testosterone and letrozole, both lumbar and femoral bone mineral density increased more slowly than in the placebo arm without reaching a statistically significant change from baseline during therapy [24]. Furthermore, in the letrozole arm, a delay in vertebral growth and maturation has been demonstrated [24]. For these reasons, as well as for the paucity of data obtained in small samples, the use of aromatase inhibitors in boys with DP is not recommended at the moment.

### *Gonadotropins*

In patients with HH, induction of puberty can be achieved with gonadotropin therapy (table 1). The most used regimen is based first on hCG followed by FSH. hCG stimulates Leydig cells leading to the increase in both intratesticular and circulating testosterone levels. The treatment with hCG alone is able to induce virilization, to improve hypogonadism-related symptoms and, in some patients, to stimulate spermatogenesis. Co-administration of FSH is required to induce spermatogenesis in patients who are not responding to hCG alone. hCG is purified from the urine of pregnant women and administered intramuscularly at doses ranging from 1,000 to 2,000 IU 2–3 times a week. FSH is available as urine-derived human menopausal gonadotropin (hMG), highly purified FSH and, more recently, as recombinant human FSH (rhFSH). Whereas hMG is a preparation containing FSH with variable traces of hCG, rhFSH and highly purified FSH have been introduced for providing preparations with pure FSH-like action. The dose usually employed ranges between 75 and 150 IU s.c. 2–3 times a week. Also recombinant hCG and LH are available,

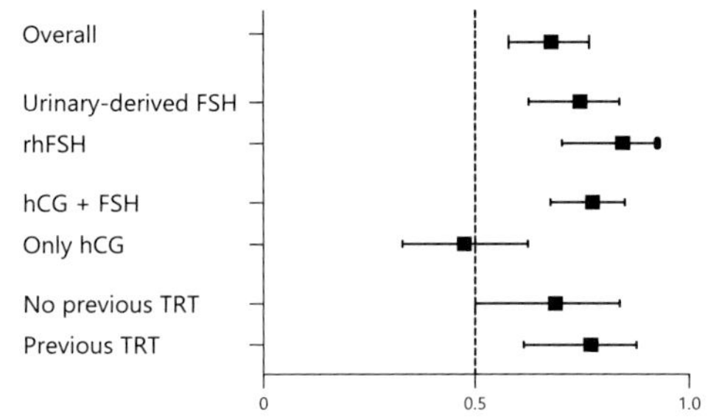


| | Studies, n | Subjects, n | Event rate | LL | UL | p |
|---|---|---|---|---|---|---|
| Overall | 26 | 445 | 0.68 | 0.58 | 0.77 | 0.001 |
| Urinary-derived FSH | 10 | 214 | 0.75 | 0.63 | 0.84 | <0.0001 |
| rhFSH | 4 | 58 | 0.85 | 0.71 | 0.93 | <0.0001 |
| hCG + FSH | 17 | 292 | 0.78 | 0.68 | 0.85 | <0.0001 |
| Only hCG | 8 | 143 | 0.47 | 0.33 | 0.62 | 0.742 |
| No previous TRT | 7 | 71 | 0.69 | 0.50 | 0.82 | 0.05 |
| Previous TRT | 12 | 128 | 0.77 | 0.62 | 0.88 | 0.001 |

**Fig. 4.** Cumulative rates (with 95% confidence intervals) of appearance of at least one spermatozoon in the semen upon gonadotropin therapy in men with prepubertal-onset HH, overall and according to different possible predictors. LL = Lower limit of the confidence interval; UL = upper limit of the confidence interval.

but their efficacy in inducing spermatogenesis has not yet been systematically studied. A classical scheme of therapy consists in starting subcutaneous injections of hCG with a dosage of 1,000 IU 2–3 times weekly for 6 months. If sperm count remains below 10 million/ml without the achievement of pregnancy, FSH is added at a dosage 75 IU s.c. every other day, which can be increased to 150 IU. Unlike with testosterone therapy, gonadotropins increase testis volume. Since low testis volume in DP boys can cause psychological distress, gonadotropin therapy can be of help in boys suffering from this physical flaw. Even more importantly, treatment with gonadotropins can induce development of testicular structures, allowing spermatogenesis. A recent meta-analysis [25] – considering all the studies that evaluated achievement of spermatogenesis with gonadotropin therapy in azoospermic HH adults – showed that 75% of subjects achieve spermatogenesis during gonadotropin treatment and, among them, significantly lower results are achieved among those who had a prepubertal onset of HH (68% achieved spermatogenesis vs. 84% in studies with a mixed population of pre- and postpubertal onset of HH). A prepubertal deficiency of pituitary gonadotropins prevents the testis from undergoing a correct and complete development, thus negatively affecting its spermatogenetic potential. It has been demonstrated that each Sertoli cell can support, in their differentiation and development, a finite number of germ cells. Hence, a decrease in Sertoli cell representation in spermatic tubules (because of the lack of stimulation in the appropriate time window) can justify an impaired spermatogenesis. Accordingly, Liu et al. [26] demonstrated better fertility outcomes in those subjects who underwent previous treatment with gonadotropins. Hence, early induction of spermatogenesis may be of help in increasing probability and reducing the time required for sperm production once fertility is required. Figure 4 shows the results of a meta-analysis of studies considering prepubertal-onset HH subjects with azoospermia who underwent gonadotropin therapy for achieving fertility. Overall, the percentage of subjects reaching spermatogenesis with gonadotropin treatment is 68%. When considering separately subjects who were treated with hCG, associated with urinary-derived or recombinant FSH, no significant difference was found in rates of achievement of sperm in semen (Q = 1.46; p = 0.227), thus suggesting that in HH males using preparations with pure FSH action, rather than hMG, does not aid in producing significantly better results. This is particularly important considering that rhFSH costs more than twice what hMG costs. No difference in reaching sperm in semen was found also when considering separately those men who were previously treated with testosterone or those who had never undergone TRT (Q = 0.78; p = 0.376). Hence, HH boys can be treated with testosterone that, whatever the preparation, has a more convenient posology than gonadotropins, without negatively affecting their future possibility of achieving fertility. When comparing studies in which only hCG was used for inducing spermatogenesis in prepubertal-onset HH men with those using combined hCG and FSH therapy, a significantly greater success rate was achieved in the latter (Q = 11.2; p = 0.001). Data from animal models show that there is a prepubertal window when FSH can induce Sertoli cell proliferation in immature testis [27]. In line with this hypothesis, FSH treatment in adolescents with prepubertal-onset HH, used as a priming before adding hCG, has been demonstrated to be able to induce inhibin B increase, testis growth and pubertal development as well as achievement of spermatogenesis [28]. In addition, in a recent randomized open-label clinical trial, 13 HH subjects were treated with GnRH alone or after a pretreatment with recombinant FSH [29]. In the arm undergoing FSH pretreatment in comparison with subjects treated with GnRH alone, a maturation of testis histology and a higher improvement in sperm count was observed. These effects have been ascribed to an FSH-mediated proliferation and maturation of Sertoli cells, which are lost in subjects with gonadotropin deficiency.

### *Gonadotropin-Releasing Hormone*

GnRH can be used alternatively to gonadotropins in inducing puberty and/or fertility in HH subjects (table 1). It stimulates the release of LH and FSH from the pituitary and, for this reason, its use is confined to those patients whose pituitary gonadotropic cells are functioning [25], as documented by GnRH test. GnRH must be administered in a pulsatile fashion in order to mimic the activity of the hypothalamic pulse generator. The dosage required for stimulating a pulsatile secretion of gonadotropins is the intravenous or subcutaneous administration of 25 ng/kg of GnRH at intervals of 90–120 min [4]. Dosage must be titrated on the basis of testosterone, LH and FSH levels. This therapy allows for full development of testicular function, both for spermatogenesis and steroidogenesis, as demonstrated by a recent meta-analysis considering all the available studies on HH subjects treated with GnRH [25]. Pulsatile GnRH is not a routinely employed therapy because administration through portable pumps is not practical and well tolerated, and it does not present any advantage in comparison with gonadotropin therapy [4].

### *Kisspeptin and Neurokinin B*

Other products that can be theoretically used for DP treatment are kisspeptin or NKB agonists, which, however, are still not available for clinical use [see ref. 30 for review].

Both native and synthetic kisspeptin agonists have been studied. Native forms have full biological activity but low molecular stability, whereas synthetic compounds are modifications of native forms made for providing resistance to degradation and for improving pharmacokinetics. These compounds bind to kisspeptin receptor (GPR54), thus stimulating GnRH and consequently gonadotropin release. Although they have still not been studied in DP, data on their use in type 2 diabetes mellitus-associated HH have been published [see ref. 30 for review]. At the moment, a clinical trial administering kisspeptin (kisspeptin 112–121; 0.24 nmol/kg) to DP boys and girls in order to determine if the pubertal delay is self-resolved or permanent is ongoing (https://clinicaltrials.gov/ct2/show/NCT01438034?ter<m = testosterone+puberty+male&rank = 4). In this study, which started enrolling patients in August 2011 and finished in October 2014, follow-up data of each participant will be collected every 6 months until they reach 18 years of age.

NKB is involved in GnRH-gonadotropin secretion. TACR3, the NKB receptor, is not expressed by GnRH neurons [see ref. 30 for review] but it is by KNDy cells, so NKB is hypothesized to act in an autocrine or paracrine manner to enhance secretion of kisspeptin, thus indirectly affecting GnRH-gonadotropin secretion [see ref. 30 for review]. Few NKB agonists, e.g. senktide and [MePhe7]NKB, have been developed for having a higher stability and affinity for TACR3 than the native molecule [see ref. 30 for review]. Although they still have not been tested in clinical studies, NKB agonists could potentially be a new therapeutic option for the treatment of DP.

## References


1 Morelli A, Marini M, Mancina R, Luconi M, Vignozzi L, Fibbi B, Filippi S, Pezzatini A, Forti G, Vannelli GB, Maggi M: Sex steroids and leptin regulate the 'first Kiss' (KiSS 1/G-protein-coupled receptor 54 system) in human gonadotropin-releasing-hormone-secreting neuroblasts. J Sex Med 2008;5:1097–1113.

2 Morelli A, Fibbi B, Marini M, Silvestrini E, De Vita G, Chavalmane AK, Vignozzi L, Filippi S, Forti G, Vannelli GB, Maggi M: Dihydrotestosterone and leptin regulate gonadotropin-releasing hormone (GnRH) expression and secretion in human GnRH-secreting neuroblasts. J Sex Med 2009;6:397–407.

3 Castellano JM, Navarro VM, Fernandez-Fernandez R, Nogueiras R, Tovar S, Roa J, Vazquez MJ, Vigo E, Casanueva FF, Aguilar E, Pinilla L, Dieguez C, Tena-Sempere M: Changes in hypothalamic KiSS1 system and restoration of pubertal activation of the reproductive axis by kisspeptin in undernutrition. Endocrinology 2005;146:3917–3925.
4 Maggi M, Buvat J: Standard operating procedures: pubertas tarda/delayed puberty – male. J Sex Med 2013;10:285–293.
5 Dunkel L, Quinton R: Transition in endocrinology: induction of puberty. Eur J Endocrinol 2014;170: R229–R239.
6 Sedlmeyer IL, Palmert MR: Delayed puberty: analysis of a large case series from an academic center. J Clin Endocrinol Metab 2002;87:1613–1620.
7 Coutant R, Biette-Demeneix E, Bouvattier C, Bouhours-Nouet N, Gatelais F, Dufresne S, Rouleau S, Lahlou N: Baseline inhibin B and anti-Mullerian hormone measurements for diagnosis of hypogonadotropic hypogonadism (HH) in boys with delayed puberty. J Clin Endocrinol Metab 2010;95: 5225–5232.
8 Raivio T, Falardeau J, Dwyer A, Quinton R, Hayes FJ, Hughes VA, Cole LW, Pearce SH, Lee H, Boepple P, Crowley WF Jr, Pitteloud N: Reversal of idiopathic hypogonadotropic hypogonadism. N Engl J Med 2007;357:863–873.
9 Sidhoum VF, Chan YM, Lippincott MF, Balasubramanian R, Quinton R, Plummer L, Dwyer A, Pitteloud N, Hayes FJ, Hall JE, Martin KA, Boepple PA, Seminara SB: Reversal and relapse of hypogonadotropic hypogonadism: resilience and fragility of the reproductive neuroendocrine system. J Clin Endocrinol Metab 2014;99:861–870.
10 Corona G, Rastrelli G, Vignozzi L, Maggi M: Emerging medication for the treatment of male hypogonadism. Expert Opin Emerg Drugs 2012;17:239–259.
11 Corona G, Rastrelli G, Forti G, Maggi M: Update in testosterone therapy for men. J Sex Med 2011;8:639–654.
12 Gupta MK, Brown DC, Faiman C, Kelnar CJ, Wu FC: Effect of low-dose testosterone treatment on androgen regulated proteins prostate specific antigen and sex hormone binding globulin in short prepubertal boys: lack of initiation of puberty. J Pediatr Endocrinol Metab 2003;16:55–62.
13 Butler GE, Sellar RE, Walker RF, Hendry M, Kelnar CJ, Wu FC: Oral testosterone undecanoate in the management of delayed puberty in boys: pharmacokinetics and effects on sexual maturation and growth. J Clin Endocrinol Metab 1992;75:37–44.
14 Ahmed SF, Tucker P, Mayo A, Wallace AM, Hughes IA: Randomized, crossover comparison study of the short-term effect of oral testosterone undecanoate and intramuscular testosterone depot on linear growth and serum bone alkaline phosphatase. J Pediatr Endocrinol Metab 2004;17:941–950.
15 De Sanctis V, Vullo C, Urso L, Rigolin F, Cavallini A, Caramelli K, Daugherty C, Mazer N: Clinical experience using the Androderm testosterone transdermal system in hypogonadal adolescents and young men with beta-thalassemia major. J Pediatr Endocrinol Metab 1998;11:891–900.
16 Mayo A, Macintyre H, Wallace AM, Ahmed SF: Transdermal testosterone application: pharmacokinetics and effects on pubertal status, short-term growth, and bone turnover. J Clin Endocrinol Metab 2004;89:681–687.
17 Rogol AD, Swerdloff RS, Reiter EO, Ross JL, Zum-Brunnen TL, Pratt GA, Brennan JJ, Benesh J, Kan-Dobrosky N, Miller MG: A multicenter, open-label, observational study of testosterone gel (1%) in the treatment of adolescent boys with Klinefelter syndrome or anorchia. J Adolesc Health 2014;54:20–25.
18 Zacharin MR, Warne GL: Treatment of hypogonadal adolescent boys with long acting subcutaneous testosterone pellets. Arch Dis Child 1997;76:495–499.
19 Crowne EC, Wallace WH, Moore C, Mitchell R, Robertson WH, Holly JM, Shalet SM: Effect of low dose oxandrolone and testosterone treatment on the pituitary-testicular and GH axes in boys with constitutional delay of growth and puberty. Clin Endocrinol (Oxf) 1997;46:209–216.
20 Wilson DM, McCauley E, Brown DR, Dudley R: Oxandrolone therapy in constitutionally delayed growth and puberty. Bio-Technology General Corporation Cooperative Study Group. Pediatrics 1995; 96:1095–1100.
21 Albanese A, Kewley GD, Long A, Pearl KN, Robins DG, Stanhope R: Oral treatment for constitutional delay of growth and puberty in boys: a randomised trial of an anabolic steroid or testosterone undecanoate. Arch Dis Child 1994;71:315–317.
22 Crowne EC, Wallace WH, Moore C, Mitchell R, Robertson WR, Shalet SM: Degree of activation of the pituitary-testicular axis in early pubertal boys with constitutional delay of growth and puberty determines the growth response to treatment with testosterone or oxandrolone. J Clin Endocrinol Metab 1995;80:1869–1875.
23 Dunkel L, Wickman S: Novel treatment of delayed male puberty with aromatase inhibitors. Horm Res 2002;57:44–52.

24 Hero M, Toiviainen-Salo S, Wickman S, Mäkitie O, Dunkel L: Vertebral morphology in aromatase inhibitor-treated males with idiopathic short stature or constitutional delay of puberty. J Bone Miner Res 2010;25:1536–1543.
25 Rastrelli G, Corona G, Mannucci E, Maggi M: Factors affecting spermatogenesis upon gonadotropin-replacement therapy: a meta-analytic study. Andrology 2014;2:794–808.
26 Liu PY, Baker HW, Jayadev V, Zacharin M, Conway AJ, Handelsman DJ: Induction of spermatogenesis and fertility during gonadotropin treatment of gonadotropin-deficient infertile men: predictors of fertility outcome. J Clin Endocrinol Metab 2009;94: 801–808.
27 Majumdar SS, Sarda K, Bhattacharya I, Plant TM: Insufficient androgen and FSH signaling may be responsible for the azoospermia of the infantile primate testes despite exposure to an adult-like hormonal milieu. Hum Reprod 2012;27:2515–2525.
28 Raivio T, Toppari J, Perheentupa A, McNeilly AS, Dunkel L: Treatment of prepubertal gonadotrophin-deficient boys with recombinant human follicle-stimulating hormone. Lancet 1997;350:263–264.
29 Dwyer AA, Sykiotis GP, Hayes FJ, Boepple PA, Lee H, Loughlin KR, Dym M, Sluss PM, Crowley WF Jr, Pitteloud N: Trial of recombinant follicle-stimulating hormone pretreatment for GnRH-induced fertility in patients with congenital hypogonadotropic hypogonadism. J Clin Endocrinol Metab 2013;98: E1790–E1795.
30 Corona G, Rastrelli G, Maggi M: The pharmacotherapy of male hypogonadism besides androgens. Expert Opin Pharmacother 2015;16:369–387.

Mario Maggi, MD
Sexual Medicine and Andrology Unit
Department of Experimental and Clinical Biomedical Sciences Mario Serio
University of Florence
Viale Pieraccini 6, IT–50139 Florence (Italy)
E-Mail mario.maggi@unifi.it

Cappa M, Cianfarani S, Ghizzoni L, Loche S, Maghnie M (eds): Advanced Therapies in Pediatric Endocrinology and Diabetology. Endocr Dev. Basel, Karger, 2016, vol 30, pp 79–97 (DOI: 10.1159/000439333)

# Long-Acting Growth Hormone: An Update

Paul H. Saenger · Jorge Mejia-Corletto

Division of Pediatric Endocrinology, Department of Pediatrics, Winthrop University Hospital, Mineola, New York, N.Y., USA

**Abstract**

After the introduction of recombinant human growth hormone (rhGH) in 1985, a myriad of children and adults have benefited from its growth-promoting and metabolic effects. Nowadays, current therapeutic regimens rely on daily subcutaneous GH injections that could be burdensome and inconvenient to pediatric patients. As expected with any long-term parenteral pharmacological treatment, these daily regimens may promote nonadherence, poor compliance, treatment abandonment and/or suboptimal clinical outcomes. In order to improve patient and caregiver acceptance of proposed regimens, simplified dosing schedules could potentially aid in reducing poor compliance and maximize the therapeutic end results. Long-acting GH formulations have been designed and perfected over the last two decades, and currently there are several formulations in advanced stages of research as a reasonable attempt to improve patient's adherence to GH treatment. A long-acting GH preparation allowing for reduced injection frequency is likely to improve treatment adherence and to decrease the distress and inconvenience associated with daily injections. This review presents an update about the status of current and recent efforts that have enabled the formulation of sustained-release, long-acting rhGH as it has been longed for many years in the pediatric endocrinology field.



## Historic Perspective and Physiological Rationale for Growth Hormone Therapy

In the late 1950s, Raben [1] was able to isolate and subsequently purify growth hormone (GH) from cadaveric human pituitaries. However, its clinical use was restricted due to limited availability of supplies and the main beneficiaries were a limited number of children with GH deficiency (GHD). Many attempts to synthesize the human GH (hGH) protein failed until 1979, when recombinant DNA technology became the standard to produce a large supply of the native, 22-kDa, 191-amino-acid-long hGH, and hundreds of thousands patients benefited from the growth-promoting and metabolic effects of hGH on the human body.

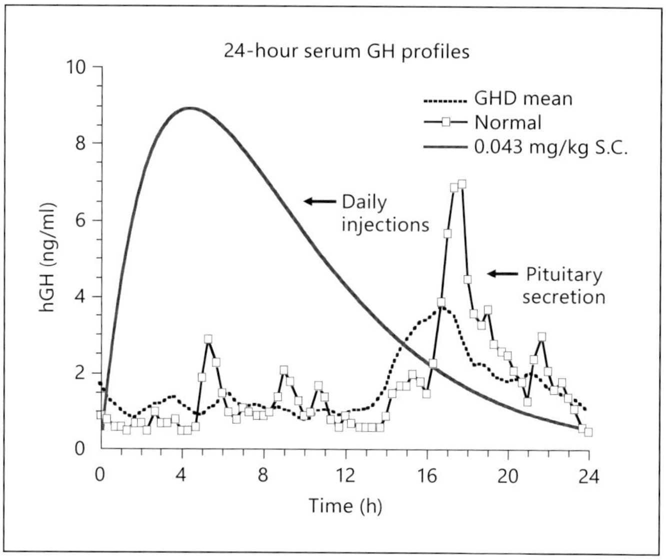


**Fig. 1.** Physiological pulsatile GH release contrasted with GHD and GH replacement therapy with daily subcutaneous injections.

*Is Daily Recombinant Human Growth Hormone Physiological?*

Physiologically, GH is synthesized by the somatotroph cells in the anterior pituitary gland under hypothalamic control via GH-releasing hormone (GHRH) and ghrelin stimuli (both secretagogues) and a negative feedback system through somatostatin and insulin-like growth factor 1 (IGF-1). There is a complex regulatory system that controls the pulsatile release of GH bursts into the peripheral circulation approximately every 3 h (6–8 discrete pulses daily) mainly during slow-wave sleep. Even though GHRH and somatostatin have been recognized as the main modulators of this axis, there are a number of other key players that seem to be important to achieve the optimal biological effects of this hormone, including ghrelin, glucocorticoids, thyroid hormones, nutritional and pubertal status, bone age as well as other metabolic and age-related mechanisms [2]. This complex physiological regulation system has not only a theoretical interest but also clinical implications. None of the previously or currently recommended GH regimens to treat GHD in pediatric or adult populations are actually physiological (fig. 1). Nevertheless, these nonphysiological replacement therapies have many years of safety data records and promote linear growth without major safety concerns.

The early regimens for GH therapy which included 2 or 3 intramuscular injections weekly were rapidly replaced by a more convenient and tolerable regimen of daily subcutaneous injections. Evidence from multiple studies has demonstrated that daily subcutaneous injections are at least as effective to generate IGF-1 production and promote linear growth as earlier attempts to treat GHD patients with twice or thrice intramuscular injections, continuous intravenous infusions or even more 'physiological' pulsatile replacement [3, 4]. Nevertheless, the efficacy and tolerability of the current standard regimen also implies adherence concerns.

*Adherence to Growth Hormone Therapy: Poor Compliance Reduces Treatment Outcomes*

Since recombinant hGH (rhGH) became available to treat GHD patients, it has been clear that clinical outcomes rely significantly upon therapeutic adherence to the proposed regimens. The efficacy and long-term outcomes from any medical therapy depend upon multiple factors, including compliance to the regimen; the presence of clinical objective and/or subjective improvement; occurrence and tolerability of possible adverse effects from the therapy; financial burden, and cultural and/or religious beliefs, among many others. There are many inherent difficulties in the long-term adherence to GH therapy that ultimately affect the outcomes of such therapy. Some of the identified barriers for good compliance include: the type of device used for administration (including its mechanical properties, its complexity, and the need for reconstitution or cartridge insertion), the frequency and route of administration, pain associated with injections, delays in filling medication from insurance carriers or specialty pharmacies, parental or patients' perceived benefits and formulary changes, among many others. In clinical settings, when assessing response to growth-promoting therapy, there are several ways to inquire about patient's adherence (table 1) [5], including parental or patient self-reporting of GH dosing, recall of missed doses in between clinic visits, collection of utilized vials of medication, review of device logs (records) at office visits and records from specialty pharmacies about medication possession ratios, for example. There is substantial evidence about the discordance between self-reported and recorded adherence by different methods [6, 7].

When compliance was assessed objectively by the number of GH vials requested by the family or the number of empty GH vials returned to the source, Cutfield et al. [6] found that only 34% of 177 patients aged 12.1 ± 0.6 years on GH therapy were compliant (defined as no more than one missed dose per week on average) and had a better linear growth [measured by height velocity (HV) standard deviation scores (HVSDS)] than noncompliant patients, suggesting that these methods are more reliable indicators of compliance than parental- *or* patient-based information (fig. 2) [6].

Miller [8] also demonstrated that GH compliance positively affects growth velocity Z-scores (ascertained by measuring medication possession ratios from specialty pharmacy records). According to questionnaire surveys conducted by Rosenfeld and Bakker [9] on 158 adults and 326 adolescents receiving GH, and 398 parents of children currently or previously receiving GH, 66–77% of patients were categorized as noncompliant, predominantly in the teenage years. The strongest factors associated with noncompliance were: misperceptions about the consequences of a missed GH dose; discomfort with injections; dissatisfaction with treatment results, and inadequate contact with health care providers. Even though compliance can be improved through utilization of user-friendly GH administration devices, frequent clinical

**Table 1.** Methods of measuring adherence

| Test | Advantages | Disadvantages |
|---|---|---|
| *Direct methods* | | |
| Directly observed therapy | Most accurate | Patients can hide pills in the mouth and then discard them; impractical for routine use |
| Measurement of the level of medicine or metabolite in blood | Objective | Variations in metabolism and 'white coat adherence' can give a false impression of adherence; expensive |
| Measurements of the biological marker in blood | Objective; in clinical trials, can also be used to measure placebo | Requires expensive quantitative assays and collection of bodily fluids |
| *Indirect methods* | | |
| Patient self-questionnaires, patient self-reports | Simple; inexpensive; the most useful method in the clinical setting | Susceptible to error with increases in time between visits; results are easily distorted by the patient |
| Pill counts | Objective, quantifiable and easy to perform | Data easily altered by the patient (e.g. pill dumping) |
| Rates of prescription refills | Objective; easy to obtain data | A prescription refill is not equivalent to ingestion of medication; requires a closed pharmacy system |
| Assessment of the patient's clinical response | Simple; generally easy to perform | Factors other than medication adherence can affect clinical response |
| Electronic medication monitors | Precise; results are easily quantified; tracks patterns of taking medication | Expensive; requires return visits and downloading data from medication vials |
| Measurement of physiologic markers (e.g. heart rate in patients taking β-blockers) | Often easy to perform | Marker may be absent for other reasons (e.g. increased metabolism, poor absorption or lack of response) |
| Patient diaries | Help to correct for poor recall | Easily altered by the patient |
| When the patient is a child, questionnaire for caregiver or teacher | Simple; objective | Susceptible to distortion |

Adapted from Osterberg and Blaschke [5].

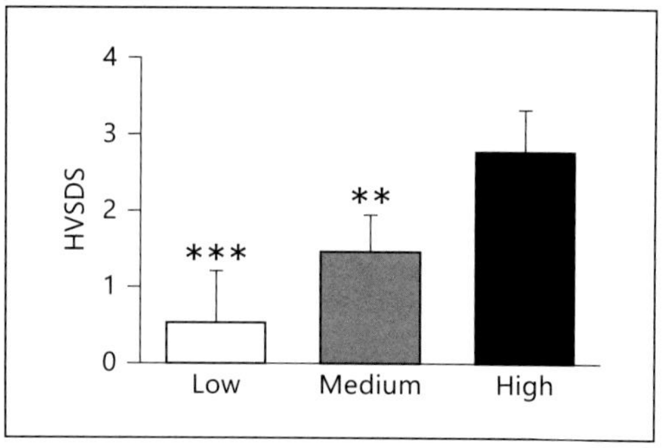


**Fig. 2.** HVSDS over 6–8 months according to the level of compliance with GH treatment: High (n = 30) missed ≤1 dose/week; medium (n = 51) missed 1–3 doses/week, and low (n = 29) missed ≥3 doses/week. Means ± SEM. ** $p < 0.01$, *** $p < 0.001$ vs. high. Reproduced with permission from Cutfield et al. [6].

**Table 2.** Strategies for improving adherence to a medication regimen

| |
|---|
| Identify poor adherence |
| Look for markers of nonadherence: missed appointments ('no shows'), lack of response to medication, missed refills |
| Ask about barriers to adherence without being confrontational |
| Emphasize the value of the regimen and the effect of adherence |
| Elicit patient's feelings about his or her ability to follow the regimen and, if necessary, supports to promote adherence |
| Provide simple, clear instructions and simplify the regimen as much as possible |
| Encourage the use of a medication-taking system |
| Listen to the patient and customize the regimen in accordance with the patient's wishes |
| Obtain help from family members, friends and community services when needed |
| Reinforce desirable behavior and results when appropriate |

Adapted from Osterberg and Blaschke [5].

monitoring, parental education and improved communication with health care providers (table 2), there are inherent barriers that may still be hard to overcome when utilizing daily subcutaneous injections. Therefore, many efforts have taken place in order to improve therapeutic outcomes and reduce noncompliance rates of patients on GH, including alternative delivery routes (oral peptidyl- and nonpeptidyl GH secretagogues, or intranasal; transdermal or pulmonary GH administration), novel injection devices, or sustained-release or depot rhGH formulations with longer half-life [5, 10].

## Long-Acting or Slow-Release Growth Hormone Preparations

For many years, the pediatric endocrinology community has longed for long-acting rhGH formulations that would decrease the inconvenience of daily injections and potentially optimize patient's compliance to such therapy. Over the last two decades, this wish is getting closer to reality.

In order to address the issues with poor adherence to rhGH, improve and/or promote optimal clinical outcomes and hopefully minimize wasting of such a considerably expense drug, several strategies have been proposed and studied further, based on the premise that long-acting, extended-release or prolonged half-life hGH could certainly improve adherence to therapy. Such novey therapy modalities imply that the new formulations are more convenient and at least as safe and efficacious (noninferiority criteria) as the standard daily subcutaneous products, and the manufacturing/distribution costs do not substantially increase the financial burden for patients and/or health systems.

In the late 1970s, when the only available hGH was the one supplied by the National Pituitary Agency from cadaveric pituitaries, Lippe et al. [11] studied the utilization of an intramuscular GH gel (15%) as a depot hGH formulation twice per week with similar growth rate results compared to a thrice-weekly regimen of the standard aqueous GH solution during the 1st year, but a waning effect of growth velocity was noted in the 2nd year of treatment, even after adjusting dosing by weight.

Since then, subsequent efforts to fabricate sustained-release rhGH took place, including stabilization with zinc ($Zn^{2+}$-hGH dimeric complexes) in order to store it in secretory granules; entrapment of hGH into hydrogels, microspheres or microcapsules, or half-life extension through structural modifications or conjugation with different compounds. There have also been other enterprises that aim to increase adherence of and convenience to patients through novel injection devices or alternative delivery systems (transdermal, pulmonary or intranasal deliveries) [10], all of which have to overcome inherent difficulties in the development and production of such expensive technologies, as well to surpass the noninferiority criteria compared to the current daily injection standard of care.

### *Nutropin Depot®*

In the 1990s, a novel pharmaceutic cryogenic technology that previously allowed stabilization of low-molecular-weight drugs was applied to larger peptides, including rhGH. Johnson et al. [12] stabilized hGH into biodegradable microspheres containing polylactic-co-glycolic acid (PLGA), a polymer similar to the one in absorbable sutures, that induced elevated serum levels of hGH in monkeys and rats for 1 month.

When subsequently applied to human adults and children, the clinical benefits seemed promising. The only long-acting formulation that once became commercially available was Nutropin Depot® produced by Genentech, Inc. (San Francisco, Calif., USA). In 1999, the US Food and Drug Administration approved Nutropin Depot® as a treatment for GHD in pediatric patients. This formulation was a long-acting form of rhGH using a ProLease® (Alkermes, Inc., Cambridge, Mass., USA) depot drug delivery system comprised of micronized particles of zinc-stabilized rhGH embedded in PLGA microspheres. A multicenter, open-label trial that studied the safety and efficacy of Nutropin Depot® on 74 prepubertal children with GHD [13] showed an increased HV from 4.5 ± 2.3 to 8.4 ± 2.1 cm/year at 6 months and 7.8 ± 1.8 cm/year at 12 months, which was, however, somewhat reduced compared to the usual growth velocity improvement seen with daily subcutaneous injections. Reported injection-site-related events were common and included nodules (60%), erythema (54%), pain after injection (36%) and lipoatrophy (11%). No serious adverse events or deaths were reported. The pharmacokinetic (PK) and pharmacodynamic (PD) studies in GHD children treated with Nutropin Depot on a once-monthly (0.15 mg/kg) or bimonthly (0.075 mg/kg) regimen showed a sustained increase in GH levels for 11–14 days and

IGF-1 levels above baseline for 16–20 days. After multiple doses over 6 months, peak and trough levels showed no progressive accumulation of GH, IGF-1 or IGF binding protein-3 [14]. In 2004, Nutropin Depot was withdrawn from the market due to 'the significant resources required by both companies (Genentech and Alkermes) to continue manufacturing and commercializing the product'. Since then, several other groups have worked in the development of polymeric microparticles or microcapsules to preserve GH bioactivity and integrity. Such materials include PLGA, hydroxyethyl methacrylated dextran, monomethoxy polyethylene glycol-co-lactide and sodium hyaluronidate, among others. An inherent difficulty in the development of PLGA microspheres relies on how its chemical properties allow the protection of GH from the acidic environment that results from the microsphere degradation in live tissues and/or denaturation from its interaction with hydrophobic interphases. New materials are currently under study and further feasibility, safety and efficacy studies are required.

### *PEGylated Growth Hormone Formulations*

Another pharmacological strategy to prolong the half-life of rhGH is through structure modification via modern PEGylation technologies, whose early development began approximately four decades ago with different pharmacological compounds. PEGylation is a process that implies modification of the rhGH through conjugation with polyethylene glycol (PEG) moieties that increase hydrodynamic size of GH, which in turn increases its circulatory time through reduced clearance by filtration in the kidneys. Several PEGylated rhGH have been studied with varied PK and PD profiles that have proven to be suitable formulations for once-weekly administration regimens. Later versions of PEGylated rhGH have proven better PK/PD and efficacy profiles than earlier formulations. However, further studies are needed to explore their long-term safety and efficacy.

A phase 2 randomized, double-blind study performed in European countries in GHD adults to assess the efficacy and safety of a PEGylated rhGH named PHA-794428 reported 13 cases of injection site lipoatrophy, independent of the PEG/GH dose or IGF-1 levels, which led to discontinuation of further trials with this product [15].

Another PEGylated GH named NNC126-0083, which consists of a 43-kDa PEG moiety conjugated with rhGH at its glutamine 141 residue, has previously been shown to possess suitable PK and PD profiles for once-weekly administration in healthy or GHD adults. After analyzing the short-term safety, tolerability and PK/PD profile of single subcutaneous doses of NNC126-0083 in 31 children with GHD, no significant short-term safety or local tolerability issues were reported (including lipoatrophy); however, the observed IGF-1 profiles were not satisfactory for the four different dosing levels that were studied in this cohort [16]. Subsequently, further efforts to study this formulation were abandoned.

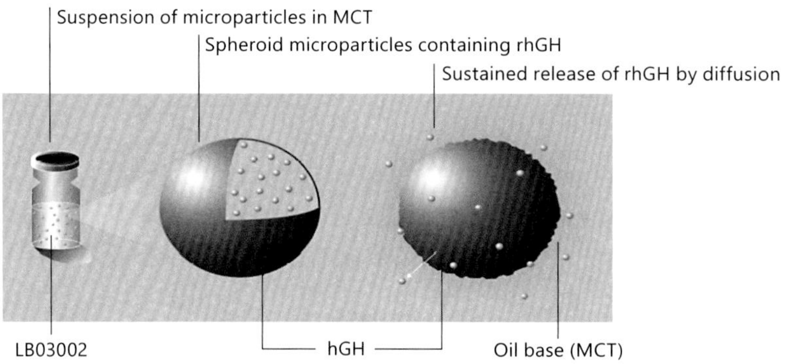


**Fig. 3.** LB03002 is a once-weekly sustained-release (depot) formulation of rhGH contained in sodium hyaluronate microparticles, which are suspended in medium-chain triglycerides (MCT) before injection. Reproduced with permission from Lee [31].

Currently, the only commercially available PEGylated rhGH is Jintrolong®, which was developed and marketed in China by GeneScience Pharmaceuticals Co., Ltd. (Changchun, China). In December 2014, recruitment was started for a phase 4, open-label trial for treatment of GHD children in the Chinese pediatric population (ClinicalTrials.gov: NCT02314676).

One of the major drawbacks of PEGylated drug products in pediatric populations is a safety concern, which originated from repeated-dose toxicity studies in cynomolgus monkeys receiving PEG moieties greater than 40 kDa for at least 6 weeks that have shown cellular vacuolation in reticuloendothelial cells, kidney tubules and also choroid plexus epithelial cells. This led to a recent warning issued by the European Medicines Agency (EMA) in 2012 [17]. The role and significance of these immunohistochemical findings that have confirmed the presence of intracytoplasmic vacuoles containing PEG in macrophages and histiocytes (presumptively as a physiological mechanism to remove foreign bodies) are yet to be determined, and it is unclear whether these are actually mechanisms operating in pediatric patients receiving PEGylated drug products, including PEG-hGH.

### *LB03002*

In 2005, Kim et al. [18] developed a sustained-release injectable rhGH named LB030002 (LG Life Sciences, Seoul, Republic of Korea) that utilized microparticles consisting of GH incorporated into a matrix of sodium hyaluronidate and lecithin dispersed in an oil base of medium-chain triglycerides (fig. 3). Worldwide phase 2 and phase 3 trials have been conducted by LG Life Sciences and BioPartners.

**Table 3.** Auxological data from the KIGS database [30] versus LB03002 [20]

| Parameter | LB03002 | KIGS |
|---|---|---|
| Age, years | 7.82±2.5 | 7.10±3.30 |
| Bone age, years | 4.35±2.2 | 5.10±3.00 |
| HV, cm/year | | |
| Baseline | 2.69±1,1 | 4.90±2.00 |
| Month 12 | 11.63±2.6 | 9.10±2.70 |
| Height SDS | | |
| Baseline | –4.34±1.8 | –3.50±1.10 |
| Month 12 | –3.06±1.5 | –2.60±1.10 |

The PK/PD profiling studies demonstrated that LB03002 was suitable to become a once-weekly rhGH injectable product in adults and children [19]. In a randomized, controlled, multicenter phase 2/3a study in European countries to explore the optimal LB03002 dose to stimulate adequate long-term longitudinal growth and to establish the long-term safety profile of the compound, we showed that a once-weekly LB03002 regimen at doses of 0.5 and 0.7 mg/kg/week were as safe and effective to treat GHD, GH-naïve children as daily GH therapy of GHD children. The 1st-year growth velocity was approximately 12 cm/year for the 0.5 and 0.7 mg/kg/week LB03002 doses and 9.7 cm/year for the 0.2 mg/kg/week LB03002 dose, compared with approximately 12 cm/year for 0.03 mg/kg/day GH, which was higher than that previously reported for the study with Nutropin Depot, where 1st-year growth velocity was 7.9 cm/year for the highest dose examined and no daily GH comparator was included. When compared to the Pfizer International Growth Database KIGS (auxological data from approximately 60,000 patients on GH therapy from more than 50 countries over the last two decades), LB03002 on a once-weekly regimen showed no inferiority at 12 months of treatment and similar height SDS improvement compared to daily rhGH injections (table 3).

A recent phase 3, multinational, randomized, open-label trial compared 91 children treated with once-weekly LB03002 with 87 children on standard therapy with daily GH [20]. This is the first report of a global phase 3 clinical trial of efficacy and safety of a long-acting GH formulation for treatment of GHD children (fig. 4). During the 1st year of treatment, HV (mean ± SD) was 11.63 ± 2.60 cm/year in the LB03002 group and 11.97 ± 3.09 cm/year in the daily GH group. Noninferiority of LB03002 treatment versus daily GH was demonstrated, with least square mean difference in HV between LB03002 and daily GH of –0.43 cm/year (99% confidence interval –1.45 to 0.60 cm/year). In the 2nd year, HV was lower, as is anticipated with any GH therapy, yet remained in line with 2nd-year growth rates published for other GH products. Treatment with LB03002 led to increased IGF-1 levels toward the normal range. Expected growth rates were maintained for 24 months, and patients retained a sustained growth potential without excessive bone maturation. LB03002 was well tolerated,

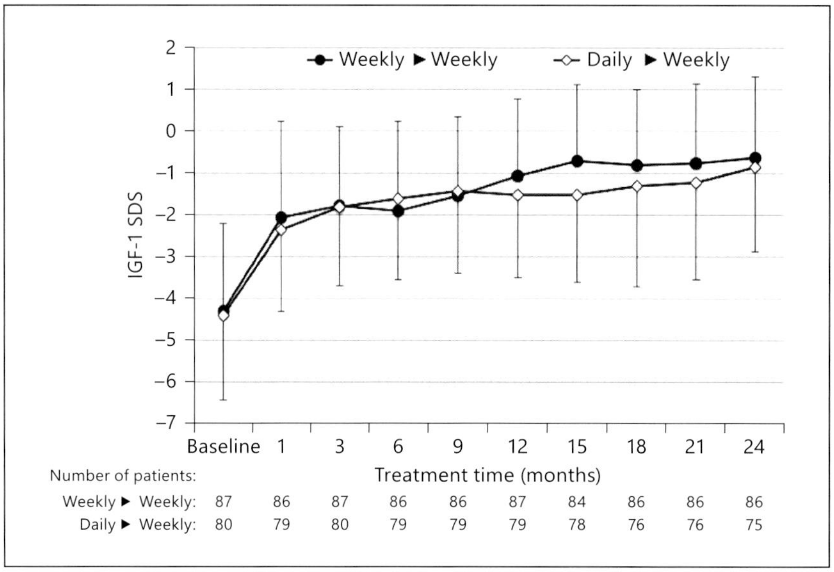


**Fig. 4.** IGF-1 SDS over time in GHD children treated with either once-weekly LB03002 (weekly) or daily GH (daily) for the first 12 months, followed by once-weekly LB03002 for both groups from months 12 to 24. Means ± SD of all patients who entered the extension study. Reproduced with permission from Khadilkar et al. [20].

with no unexpected safety issues. No nodules or lipoatrophy were reported. Overall, this makes once-weekly LB03002 a valid candidate for long-term GH replacement in GHD children, and further studies on its efficacy and safety over more extensive time periods will be carried out. LB03002 was approved by EMA in August 2013 for the treatment of GHD in children and adults. There has been no commercial release since then. It is available in Korea.

*Protein Fusion/Conjugation Technologies*

*VRS-317*

Cleland et al. [21] produced a novel rhGH with prolonged half-life named VRS-317 (Versartis Inc., Menlo Park, Calif., USA). VRS-317 is a fusion protein consisting of rhGH and a proprietary half-life extension technology known as XTEN, which is in-licensed from Amunix Operating, Inc. (Menlo Park, Calif,, USA), formulated by fusing a sequence of hydrophilic amino acids as a head and a tail to both C- and N-terminal sequences of the rhGH (fig. 5).

VRS-317 is a fusion protein (molecular mass of 119 kDa) produced in *Escherichia coli*. The pharmacologically active portion is the rhGH domain (22 kDa), and the pharmacologically inactive domains are long chains of natural hydrophilic amino acids, designated as $XTEN_1$ and $XTEN_2$ domains. The long N-terminal $XTEN_1$ domain

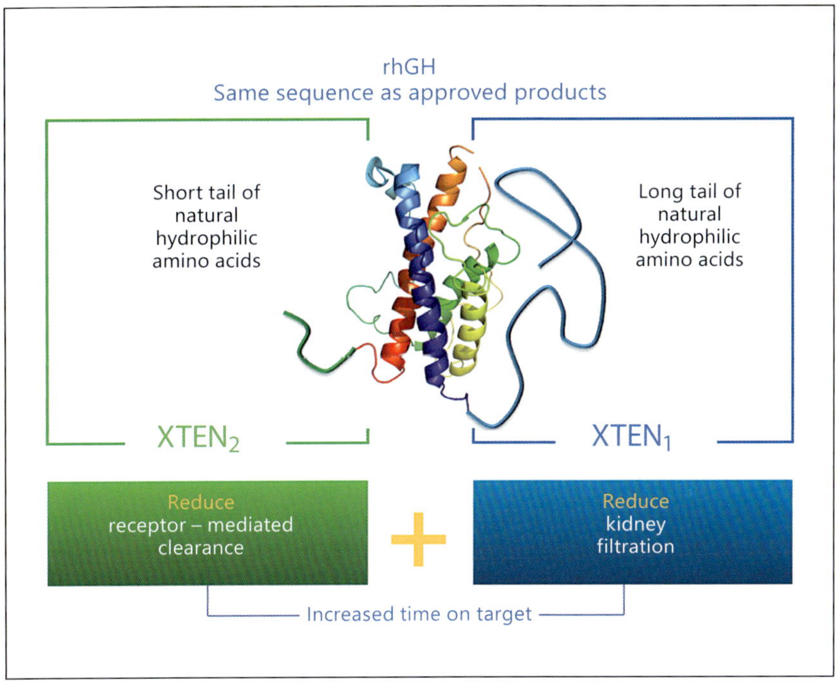


**Fig. 5.** Molecular structure of VRS-317, depicted as a fusion protein with a pharmacologically active portion (rhGH domain) and two pharmacologically inactive domains (long chains of natural hydrophilic amino acids), designated as $XTEN_1$ and $XTEN_2$ domains. $XTEN_1$ enables the extension of the half-life of rhGH by increasing its hydrodynamic size and, thereby, reducing glomerular filtration. $XTEN_2$ delays receptor-mediated clearance by decreasing receptor affinity and binding. Reproduced with permission from Bright et al. [32].

enables extension of the half-life of rhGH by increasing the hydrodynamic size of rhGH and, thereby, reducing glomerular filtration. The shorter C-terminal $XTEN_2$ delays receptor-mediated clearance by decreasing receptor affinity and binding. In monkeys, VRS-317 displayed a terminal elimination half-life of approximately 110 h. Although the in vitro potency of VRS-317 was reduced by approximately 12-fold compared with that of rhGH, the in vivo potency was increased because of the greatly prolonged exposure at target tissues. Interim results of a phase 2a study presented at the Endocrine Society's 96th Annual Meeting and Expo (ICE/ENDO 2014) demonstrated that the efficacy and safety of VRS-317, when administered monthly, semimonthly and weekly in pediatric patients with GHD, are comparable to daily injections of rhGH. Subjects were randomized to VRS-317 doses of 5 mg/kg monthly, 2.5 mg/kg semimonthly or 1.15 mg/kg weekly for 6 months [22]. When HV data were compared to data for the first 12 months of treatment in age-matched GHD children in the KIGS database (Pfizer International Growth Database), annualized mean HV at 6 months was 7.6 compared to 8.4 cm/year (historical controls) in the weekly arm, 8.7 compared to 8.3 cm/year (historical controls) in the semimonthly arm, and 7.9

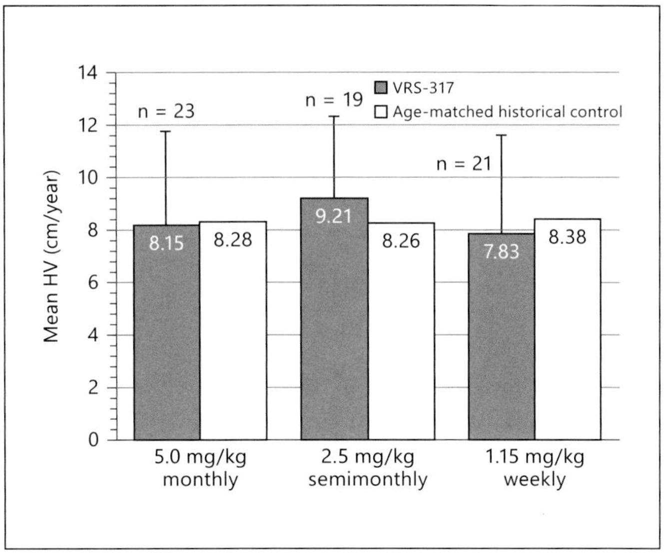


**Fig. 6.** Annualized growth velocity during a phase 2a trial with VRS-317 of 64 prepubertal children with GHD naïve to rhGH randomized into three dosing arms to evaluate 5.0 mg/kg monthly, 2.5 mg/kg semimonthly or 1.15 mg/kg weekly (cumulative dose of 30 mg/kg/6 months for all). Reproduced with permission from Bright et al. [22].

compared to 8.3 cm/year (historical controls) in the monthly arm (fig. 6). There was no statistically significant difference between any of the three dosing frequencies tested, and VRS-317 was safe and well tolerated in naïve, prepubertal GHD children. There was a significant and expected increase in IGF-1 levels versus baseline in patients treated with VRS-317. Additionally, IGF-1 responses were maintained for the duration of all three dosing intervals and there is no evidence of IGF-1 accumulation. There were no drug-related serious adverse events or unexpected adverse events. Neither nodules nor lipoatrophy was observed at any of the more than 1,500 injection sites monitored as part of the phase 2a study. A 6-month extension showed an increase in annualized HV in the subset of patients for whom the dose was increased from a weekly dose of 1.15 mg/kg in the phase 2a trial to a semimonthly dose of 3.5 mg/kg in the extension study (from 7.5 cm/year in the first 6 months to 9.3 cm/year in the second 6 months). In January 2015, a randomized, open-label, phase 3 study was started to be conducted in the United States, Western Europe and Canada using a reformulated drug.

*MOD-4023*

Another novel rhGH with prolonged half-life was developed by conjugation of a carboxyl-terminus peptide (CTP) from human chorionic gonadotropin (hCG) to rhGH (Prolor Biotech Inc., Nes Ziona, Israel). Previous studies indicated that fusing the CTP of the hCG β-subunit to human follitropin (FSHβ), hCGα, TSHβ or to erythropoietin did not affect assembly, secretion, receptor binding affinity or in vitro bioactivity. However, the in vivo potency and circulatory half-lives of the proteins containing CTP were substantially increased [23]. Considering that the CTP on its β subunit accounts for the prolonged half-life of hCG when compared to luteinizing hormone, a

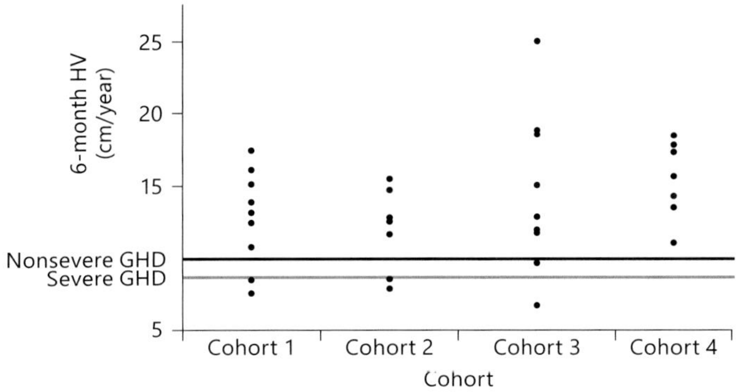


| Cohort | Dose | hGH content | n | Mean (cm/year) | SD |
|---|---|---|---|---|---|
| Cohort 1 | 0.25 mg/kg/w MOD-4023 | 0.18 mg/kg/w | 9 | 13.48 | 2.71 |
| Cohort 2 | 0.48 mg/kg/w MOD-4023 | 0.35 mg/kg/w | 9 | 12.25 | 2.64 |
| Cohort 3 | 0.66 mg/kg/w MOD-4023 | 0.48 mg/kg/w | 10 | 14.37 | 5.26 |
| Cohort 4 | 0.034 mg/kg/d Genotropin | 0.21 mg/kg/w | 7 | 15.46 | 2.68 |

**Fig. 7.** A randomized, comparator-controlled phase 2 study was conducted in 56 prepubertal, naïve GHD children receiving one of three MOD-4023 doses as once-weekly regimen (0.25, 0.48 and 0.66 mg/kg/week) or daily hGH (34 µg/kg/day) as comparator arm in subcutaneous injections [24]. Mean annualized HV at 6 months ranged from 12.25 to 14.37 cm vs. ~15.46 cm in the comparator group receiving daily subcutaneous rhGH. d = Day; w = week. Definition of severe and nonsevere GHD as per Ranke et al. [25].

new formulation of a chimeric hGH named MOD-4023 was created by fusing one copy of CTP to the N-terminal peptide and two copies of CTP to the C-terminal peptide of the native rhGH.

Based on the PK/PD and efficacy results of phase 2 and 3 clinical trials, this modification confers extended half-life suitable for a once-weekly dosing regimen for the treatment of adults and children [24] with GHD. In the phase 2 trial in children with GHD treated with MOD-4023, mean HV at 6 months ranged from 12.25 to 14.37 cm/year, compared to mean HV of 15.46 cm/year from the comparator cohort receiving daily subcutaneous rhGH (fig. 7).

*ACP-001*

Since 2002, a new technology named TransCon was developed and matured in order to extend the half-life of several proteins, peptides and other molecules, including rhGH (Ascendis Pharma A/S, Copenhagen, Denmark). A formulation named ACP-001 consists of PEGylated rhGH as an inactive prodrug linked to a TransCon carrier

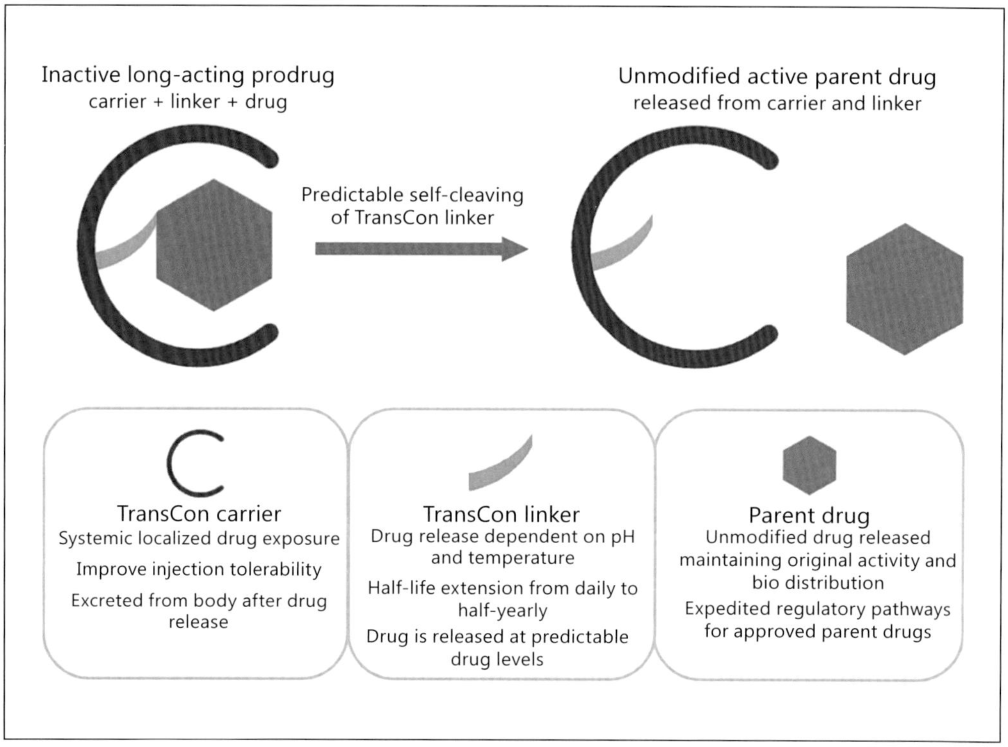


**Fig. 8.** Pharmaceutical principle of TransCon technology. An inactive long-acting prodrug consisting of the following triad: a TransCon carrier that improves tolerability and is excreted from the body after GH release; a TransCon linker that binds the parent drug to the carrier and extends the half-life of the rhGH, and the parent drug (rhGH) that is cleaved from the linker at predetermined rates governed by physiological pH and temperature conditions. Adapted from Ascendis Pharma (http://www.ascendispharma.com/technology).

that, after absorption into the bloodstream, acts as a circulating reservoir that releases GH over a predictable amount of time governed by physiological pH and temperature conditions (fig. 8).

A phase 2 trial in adults with GHD showed a PK/PD profile suitable for once-weekly subcutaneous administration and dose-dependent IGF-1 responses. No lipoatrophy was reported and only mild injection site reactions were noted. An ongoing phase 2 pediatric study is being conducted to investigate the safety, tolerability, PK/PD profile and efficacy of TransCon GH in the treatment of GH-naïve prepubertal patients with GHD. The study is a 6-month multicenter, randomized study comparing three dose levels of TransCon GH (0.14, 0.21 and 0.30 mg rhGH/kg/week), administered once per week, to an active control (0.21 mg rhGH/kg/week), administered as a daily injection. Interim results on press coverage showed that among the three dosing levels administered weekly, mean HV ranged from 11.9 cm/year for the 0.14 mg/kg/week dose to 14.5 cm/year for the 0.30 mg/kg/week dose, which were comparable to 11.5

cm/year for the active comparator, daily injections of Genotropin® at 0.21 mg/kg/week. No major safety concerns have been reported and the IGF-1 profile showed dose-proportional responses for the three dose regimens analyzed (interim results on http://www.prnewswire.com/news-releases/ascendis-pharma-as-announces-positive-six-month-interim-results-from-a-phase-2-pediatric-study-of-once-weekly-transcon-growth-hormone-for-the-treatment-of-growth-hormone-deficiency-300009157.html).

*Growth Hormone-Albumin Binding Technologies*

In the late 1980s, Poznansky et al. [26] successfully created a porcine GH formulation conjugated to homologous serum albumin, with glutaraldehyde as a cross-linking agent. This GH-albumin conjugate displayed altered PK with prolonged plasma clearance compared to the native nonconjugated GH, presumptively to decrease renal filtration and excretion of GH. However, these assays failed to demonstrate a growth-promoting effect on hypophysectomized rats.

Subsequent efforts led to formulate Albutropin, a hGH fused at its N terminus with human serum albumin [27]. After subcutaneous dosing in rats, a 2-fold decrease in clearance and a 4-fold increase in plasma half-life were seen with Albutropin compared to GH. In monkeys, subcutaneous Albutropin (0.3 mg/kg) had a 6-fold longer terminal half-life and an 8-fold slower clearance than rhGH (0.3 mg/kg). Currently, there are ongoing phase 2 clinical trials for safety, tolerability and efficacy for weekly subcutaneous Albutropin named TV-1106 (TEVA Pharmaceutical Industries Ltd., Petach Tikva, Israel) in adults with GHD as well as a phase 2 safety and dose-finding study in children with GHD (ClinicalTrials.gov: NCT01811576 and NCT02092077, respectively).

A novel technology developed a modified rhGH named NNC0195-0092 (Novo Nordisk A/S, Bagsværd, Denmark) in which a noncovalent reversible albumin-binding moiety is attached to the rhGH backbone. By means of a single-point mutation on the rhGH backbone, a terminal fatty acid has been attached with noncovalent albumin-binding properties. This modification also decreased renal clearance and extended in vivo half-life. Preclinical studies did not identify any safety issues in rats and monkeys. A phase 1, randomized, single-center, placebo-controlled, double-blind, single-/multiple-dose, dose-escalation trial of 105 healthy male subjects recently published showed that NNC0195-0092 was well tolerated at all dose levels. No safety concerns or local tolerability issues were identified. A dose-dependent IGF-1 response was observed. IGF-1 profiles suggest that NNC0195-0092 may be suitable for once-weekly dosing, with a clinically relevant dose of 0.08 mg/kg/week [28]. A phase 1 trial in adults with GHD was completed in November 2013 (ClinicalTrials.gov: NCT01706783) and another phase 1 single-dose trial in children with GHD was completed in November 2014 (ClinicalTrials.gov: NCT01973244). An ongoing phase 3 trial in adults with GHD recently started recruitment of patients (ClinicalTrials.gov: NCT02229851). So far, study participants have received 4 weekly doses of NNC0195-0092. Long-term trials are necessary.

*LAPS-rhGH*
Another novel fusion technology known as LAPSCOVERY™ (long-acting protein/peptide discovery platform technology), developed by Hanmi Pharmaceutical Co., Ltd. (Seoul, Republic of Korea) allowed the formulation of a hybrid drug named LAPS-rhGH (HM10560A) consisting of rhGH fused with a hybrid Fc fragment containing partial Fc domains of human IgD and $IgG_4$ to produce a long-acting fusion protein that triggered phosphorylation of human Janus kinase 2 in B lymphocytes [29]. A phase 1 trial in healthy adults was completed. Currently, phase 2 trials are ongoing to assess safety, efficacy, tolerability and PK/PD profiles in adults with GHD receiving HM10560A, either one dose every week or every other week during a total of 24 weeks (ClinicalTrials.gov: NCT01822340).

## Conclusions

In order to maximize the growth-promoting effects and other physiological benefits from GH therapy, different innovative pharmaceutical technologies have resulted in the development of long-acting, slow-release or prolonged half-life GH formulations. These efforts are the response to well-documented therapeutic-failures or suboptimal outcomes when noncompliance or poor adherence to proposed GH regimens takes place. On the one hand, even though current standards of treatment with daily subcutaneous GH administration have been proven to improve therapeutic outcomes in patients with different pathological conditions that restrict growth rate and final adult height, daily regimens inherently imply obstacles for good compliance.

A once-per-week rhGH regimen could potentially save over 1,500 injections on a typical 5-year treatment compared to standard daily therapy and could provide greater convenience, acceptability and greater compliance compared to the current standard of care.

A summary of some of the most relevant current technologies and long-acting GH formulations are shown in table 4. As these emerging pharmaceutical technologies have been applied to preclinical and clinical settings, several lessons have been learned and some requirements need to be fulfilled in order to allow any long-acting GH formulation to be clinically and commercially successful:

(a) Comparable growth rates as those achieved with daily rhGH
(b) Small injection volume
(c) Small needle, preferably a 31-gauge needle
(d) Suitable for use with a pen device
(e) Side effect profile not worse than daily rhGH
(f) Similar stimulated IGF-1 responses as with daily rhGH
(g) Comparable prices as daily rhGH

For many years, the pediatric endocrinology community has longed for long-acting rhGH formulations that would decrease the inconvenience of daily injections and

**Table 4.** Current technologies and long-acting GH formulations

| Formulation | Manufacturer | Technology | Clinical trial status |
|---|---|---|---|
| LB03002 | LG LifeSciences/ BioPartners | Microencapsulation on hyaluronidate matrix | Completed phase 3 in children<br>Approved by EMA in Aug 2013 |
| VRS-317 | Versartis | Prolonged half-life<br>XTEN fusion protein | Ongoing phase 3 in children |
| MOD-4023 | OPKO/ Prolor Biotech | Prolonged half-life<br>CTP fusion protein | Ongoing phase 3 in adults<br>Ongoing phase 2 in children |
| ACP-001 | Ascendis Pharma | Prolonged-half life<br>Prodrug<br>TransCon fusion protein | Completed phase 2 in adults<br>Ongoing phase 2 in children |
| TV-1106/ Albutropin | TEVA | Prolonged half-life<br>Albumin fusion protein | Ongoing phase 2 in adults<br>Ongoing phase 2 in children |
| NNC0195-0092 | Novo Nordisk | Prolonged half-life<br>Noncovalent albumin binding | Completed phase 1 in adults<br>Completed phase 1 in children |
| LAPS-rhGH/ HM10560A | Hanmi | Prolonged-half life<br>Fc fragment fusion protein | Ongoing phase 2 in adults<br>No trials in children yet |

potentially optimize patient's compliance to such therapy. Over the last two decades, this wish is getting closer to reality as newer pharmaceutical technologies have been designed and improved different long-acting or sustained-release GH formulations that ultimately will improve adherence to therapeutic regimens should they demonstrate long-term efficacy, safety and affordability.

## Disclosure Statement

P.H.S. was a consultant for LG LifeSciences/BioPartners.

## References


1 Raben MS: Preparation of growth hormone from pituitaries of man and monkey. Science 1957;125:883–884.

2 Goldenberg N, Barkan A: Factors regulating growth hormone secretion in humans. Endocrinol Metab Clin North Am 2007;36:37–55.

3 Jorgensen JO, Moller N, Lauritzen T, Christiansen JS: Pulsatile versus continuous intravenous administration of growth hormone (GH) in GH-deficient patients: effects on circulating insulin-like growth factor-I and metabolic indices. J Clin Endocrinol Metab 1990;70:1616–1623.

4 Laursen T, Gravholt CH, Heickendorff L, et al: Long-term effects of continuous subcutaneous infusion versus daily subcutaneous injections of growth hormone (GH) on the insulin-like growth factor system, insulin sensitivity, body composition, and bone and lipoprotein metabolism in GH-deficient adults. J Clin Endocrinol Metab 2001;86:1222–1228.

5 Osterberg L, Blaschke T: Adherence to medication. N Engl J Med 2005;353:487–497.

6 Cutfield WS, Derraik JG, Gunn AJ, et al: Non-compliance with growth hormone treatment in children is common and impairs linear growth. PLoS One 2011;6:e16223.
7 Kapoor RR, Burke SA, Sparrow SE, et al: Monitoring of concordance in growth hormone therapy. Arch Dis Child 2008;93:147–148.
8 Miller BS, Crawford M, McNamara A, Frohnert BI: Reduced medication possession ratio is associated with lower response to growth hormone therapy (abstract). Pediatric Academic Societies' Meeting, Vancouver, 2014, abstract 750310.
9 Rosenfeld RG, Bakker B: Compliance and persistence in pediatric and adult patients receiving growth hormone therapy. Endocr Pract 2008;14:143–154.
10 Cai Y, Xu M, Yuan M, Liu Z, Yuan W: Developments in human growth hormone preparations: sustained-release, prolonged half-life, novel injection devices, and alternative delivery routes. Int J Nanomedicine 2014;9:3527–3538.
11 Lippe B, Frasier SD, Kaplan SA: Use of growth hormone-gel. Arch Dis Child 1979;54:609–613.
12 Johnson OL, Jaworowicz W, Cleland JL, et al: The stabilization and encapsulation of human growth hormone into biodegradable microspheres. Pharm Res 1997;14:730–735.
13 Reiter EO, Attie KM, Moshang T Jr, et al: A multicenter study of the efficacy and safety of sustained release GH in the treatment of naive pediatric patients with GH deficiency. J Clin Endocrinol Metab 2001;86:4700–4706.
14 Kemp SF, Fielder PJ, Attie KM, et al: Pharmacokinetic and pharmacodynamic characteristics of a long-acting growth hormone (GH) preparation (Nutropin Depot) in GH-deficient children. J Clin Endocrinol Metab 2004;89:3234–3240.
15 Touraine P, D'Souza GA, Kourides I, et al: Lipoatrophy in GH deficient patients treated with a long-acting pegylated GH. Eur J Endocrinol 2009;161:533–540.
16 de Schepper J, Rasmussen MH, Gucev Z, Eliakim A, Battelino T: Long-acting pegylated human GH in children with GH deficiency: a single-dose, dose-escalation trial investigating safety, tolerability, pharmacokinetics and pharmacodynamics. Eur J Endocrinol 2011;165:401–409.
17 European Medicines Agency: CHMP Safety Working Party's response to the PDCO regarding the use of PEGylated drug products in the paediatric population. EMA/CHMP/SWP/647258/2012, http://www.ema.europa.eu/docs/en_GB/document_library/Scientific_guideline/2012/11/WC500135123.pdf.
18 Kim SJ, Hahn SK, Kim MJ, Kim DH, Lee YP: Development of a novel sustained release formulation of recombinant human growth hormone using sodium hyaluronate microparticles. J Control Release 2005;104:323–335.
19 Peter F, Savoy C, Ji HJ, Juhasz M, Bidlingmaier M, Saenger P: Pharmacokinetic and pharmacodynamic profile of a new sustained-release GH formulation, LB03002, in children with GH deficiency. Eur J Endocrinol 2009;160:349–355.
20 Khadilkar V, Radjuk KA, Bolshova E, Saenger P, et al: 24-month use of once-weekly GH, LB03002, in prepubertal children with GH deficiency. J Clin Endocrinol Metab 2014;99:126–132.
21 Cleland JL, Geething NC, Moore JA, et al: A novel long-acting human growth hormone fusion protein (VRS-317): enhanced in vivo potency and half-life. J Pharm Sci 2012;101:2744–2754.
22 Bright G, Moore WV, Nguyen HQ, et al: Safety and efficacy results of a 6 month, randomized, multi-center trial of a novel long-acting rhGH (VRS-317) in naïve to treatment, pre-pubertal children with growth hormone deficiency (GHD) (abstract). 16th International Congress of Endocrinology and the Endocrine Society's 96th Annual Meeting and Expo (ICE/ENDO 2014), Chicago, 2014, MON-0147.
23 Fares F, Guy R, Bar-Ilan A, Felikman Y, Fima E: Designing a long-acting human growth hormone (hGH) by fusing the carboxyl-terminal peptide of human chorionic gonadotropin beta-subunit to the coding sequence of hGH. Endocrinology 2010;151:4410–4417.
24 Hart G, Zadik Z, Kradziu K, Zelinska N, Malievsky O, Iotova V, Skorodok J, Koren R, Amitzi L, Fima E: Six months follow-up pharmacokinetics and pharmacodynamics profile of once-weekly, CTP-modified human GH (MOD-4023): phase 2 dose finding study in children with GHD. 53rd Annual Meeting of the European Society of Paediatric Endocrinology, Dublin, Sept 18–20th, 2014. ESPE Abstracts 2014, P-D-1-3-163.
25 Ranke MB, Lindberg A, KIGS International Board: Observed and predicted growth responses in prepubertal children with growth disorders: guidance of growth hormone treatment by empiric variables. J Clin Endocrinol Metab 2010;95:1229–1237.
26 Poznansky MJ, Halford J, Taylor D: Growth hormone-albumin conjugates. Reduced renal toxicity and altered plasma clearance. FEBS Lett 1988;239:18–22.
27 Osborn BL, Sekut L, Corcoran M, et al: Albutropin: a growth hormone-albumin fusion with improved pharmacokinetics and pharmacodynamics in rats and monkeys. Eur J Pharmacol 2002;456:149–158.

28 Rasmussen MH, Olsen MW, Alifrangis L, Klim S, Suntum M: A reversible albumin-binding growth hormone derivative is well tolerated and possesses a potential once-weekly treatment profile. J Clin Endocrinol Metab 2014;99:E1819–E1829.
29 Kim ES, Jang do S, Yang SY, et al: Controlled release of human growth hormone fused with a human hybrid Fc fragment through a nanoporous polymer membrane. Nanoscale 2013;5:4262–4269.
30 Ranke MB, Reiter E, Price D: Idiopathic growth hormone deficiency in KIGS: selected aspects; in Ranke MB, Price DA, Reiter EO (eds): Growth Hormone Therapy in Pediatrics: 20 years of KIGS. Basel, Karger, 2007, pp 116–135.
31 Lee JE: Drug delivery systems associated with pediatric endocrinology. J Korean Soc Pediatr Endocriol 2011;16:7–12.
32 Bright GM, Moore WV, Nguyen HQ, et al: Dose response and 12 month safety and efficacy of VRS-317 in pre-pubertal children with moderate growth hormone deficiency (GHD) (abstract). Endocrine Society's 97th Annual Meeting & Expo (ENDO 2015), San Diego, 2015, LBF-026.

Paul H. Saenger, MD
Division of Pediatric Endocrinology
Department of Pediatrics
Winthrop University Hospital
101 Mineola Blvd., 2nd Floor
Mineola, New York, NY 11501 (USA)
E-Mail phsaenger@gmail.com

Cappa M, Cianfarani S, Ghizzoni L, Loche S, Maghnie M (eds): Advanced Therapies in Pediatric Endocrinology and Diabetology. Endocr Dev. Basel, Karger, 2016, vol 30, pp 98–105 (DOI: 10.1159/000439334)

# C-Type Natriuretic Peptide Analog as Therapy for Achondroplasia

Laurence Legeai-Mallet

INSERM U1163, Institut Imagine, Université Paris Descartes-Sorbonne Paris Cité, Paris, France

## Abstract

Fibroblast growth factor receptor 3 (FGFR3) is an important regulator of bone formation. Gain-of-function mutations in the *FGFR3* gene result in chondrodysplasias which include achondroplasia (ACH), the most common form of dwarfism, in which skull, appendicular and axial skeletons are affected. The skeletal phenotype of patients with ACH showed defective proliferation and differentiation of the chondrocytes in the growth plate cartilage. Both endochondral and membranous ossification processes are disrupted during development. At cellular level, *Fgfr3* mutations induce increased phosphorylation of the tyrosine kinase receptor FGFR3, which correlate with an enhanced activation of its downstream signaling pathways. Potential therapeutic strategies have emerged for ACH. Several preclinical studies have been conducted such as the C-type natriuretic peptide (CNP) analog (BMN111), intermittent parathyroid hormone injections, soluble FGFR3 therapy, and meclozine and statin treatments. Among the putative targets to antagonize FGFR3 signaling, CNP (or BMN111) is one of the most promising strategies. BMN111 acts as a key regulator of longitudinal bone growth by downregulating the mitogen-activated protein kinase pathway, which is activated as a result of a *FGFR3* gain-of-function mutation. Preclinical studies showed that BMN111 treatment led to a large improvement in skeletal parameters in $Fgfr3^{Y367C/+}$ mice mimicking ACH. In 2014, a clinical trial (phase 2) of BMN111 in pediatric patients with ACH has started. This first clinical trial marks the first big step towards real treatment for these patients.



In 1994, the research field of chondrodysplasias made significant progress with the discovery that an activating mutation in the fibroblast growth factor receptor 3 (FGFR3) gene accounts for the most common genetic form of dwarfism, achondroplasia (ACH) [1, 2]. Other activating FGFR3 mutations cause a broad clinical spectrum of chondrodysplasias ranging from hypochondroplasia, a milder clinical form of ACH, SADDAN, which is a severe ACH with developmental delay, hearing loss and acanthosis nigricans to thanatophoric dysplasia (TD), a lethal dwarfism [3].

### Clinical Characteristics of Achondroplasia

ACH patients present a disproportionate short stature, characterized by short limbs, especially the proximal segments, with a long trunk deformed by excessive lordosis and a narrow thorax. The head is large with frontal bossing and the midface is hypoplastic. The size of the craniocervical junction is reduced. Hands and fingers are short with a trident appearance [4]. Today, ACH treatment focuses on managing the symptoms and health conditions. Indeed, these patients lead independent and productive lives, and they have normal intelligence and life expectancy. However, these patients need lifelong follow-up care. Health problems commonly associated with these skeletal diseases require surgery and specific medical visits. During the first few months, cervicomedullary compression can occur due to the reduced size of the foramen magnum; recurrent otitis media is common in young patients with ACH and needs to be treated to prevent conductive hearing loss. Restrictive respiratory insufficiency could be observed due to a small chest. Spinal canal stenosis and cardiovascular complications may also be present in this disorder.

### Genetics and Physiopathology

ACH is an autosomal dominant disorder, which occurs with an estimated prevalence between 1/16,000 and 1/25,000 live births. Most of the ACH patients were found to have the same p.Gly380Arg amino acid substitution in the transmembrane domain of FGFR3. This mutation is often associated with increasing paternal age. A Gly375Cys mutation of FGFR3 also accounts for a few patients with ACH. The penetrance of these mutations is 100% [3, 4].

ACH gain-of-function mutation activates the tyrosine kinase activity of the receptor and facilitates its transautophosphorylation of key tyrosine residues in the intracellular domain and seems to induce structural modifications in the FGFR3 dimer. Experimental studies demonstrate that mutations constitutively activate FGFR3 in cellular models [5, 6]. Several signaling pathways are affected by FGFR3 activation. It has been demonstrated that the canonical mitogen-activated protein kinase (MAPK) pathway regulates many effects of FGFR3. Sustained extracellular signal-regulated kinase (ERK) 1/2 activation has been observed in the presence of ACH mutations. Other signaling pathways seem to be implicated, e.g. Sox9, Stat, Wnt/β-catenin, phosphatidylinositol-3-kinase/AKT and phospholipase Cγ pathways [7–9].

The activating mutations in ACH lead to impaired cartilage development. A severe disorganization of the growth plate was observed in the ACH and TD human fetal growth plates with a marked reduction in the hypertrophic and proliferative zones. An abnormal expression of FGFR3, STAT and p21 was observed in ACH and TD growth plates thus inducing the premature exit of proliferative cells from the cell cycle and their differentiation into hypertrophic chondrocytes [7, 10]. Aberrant activation of FGFR3 induces premature growth arrest, loss of extracellular matrices and changes in cell shape [11].

Since 1996, several *Fgfr3* mouse models have been generated. The mouse model lacking *Fgfr3* had skeletal overgrowth with an expansion of the proliferative and hypertrophic zones within the growth plate [12]. These data allowed for the conclusion that FGFR3 is a negative regulator of bone growth [13]. By contrast, the Fgfr3 mutant mice expressing an Fgfr3 point mutation corresponding to ACH and TD exhibit varying degrees of disproportionate dwarfism with skeletal anomalies [14–17].

Among them, we have generated a mouse model that consists of heterozygous $Fgfr3^{Y367C/+}$ mice ubiquitously expressing the Y367C mutation corresponding to TD type I. $Fgfr3^{Y367C/+}$ mice exhibit a severe dwarfism phenotype. The $Fgfr3^{Y367C/+}$ mice showed ~50% reduction in the length of the appendicular skeleton and ~30% reduction in the length of the axial skeleton, and displayed disproportionate short stature as observed in FGFR3-related chondrodysplasias. Computed tomography scanner analysis showed the presence of an impressive dome skull and a small snout with an anterior crossbite in $Fgfr3^{Y367C/+}$ mice that is comparable with the prominent forehead (frontal bossing) and midface hypoplasia observed in human disorders. Medullary and upper spinal cord compression due to the reduced size of the foramen magnum was visualized by magnetic resonance imaging in this mouse model confirming anomalies in cervical vertebrae [18]. These signs of cervicomedullary compression due to foramen magnum stenosis are similar to those reported in ACH children [19]. $Fgfr3^{Y367C/+}$ mice exhibit hearing loss and an inner ear defect characterized by an increased number of pillar cells [14].

Histological analysis of the distal femur epiphysis revealed growth plate disorganization with a lack of chondrocyte columnar arrangement and a delay in the formation of the secondary ossification center in the long bone. We also observed severe bone anomalies in the long bones with an important reduction in cartilage matrix mineralization and the strong defects of primary spongiosa. Anomalies of primary spongiosa were associated with an increase in osteoclast recruitment and a defect in osteoblasts at the mineralization front. Significant decreases in bone volume and trabecular thickness and number were also noted in the trabecular bone of $Fgfr3^{Y367C/+}$ mice [20]. Studying the calvaria and skull base of ACH and FGFR3-related craniosynostosis patients and $Fgfr3^{Y367C/+}$ mice, we observed abnormal cartilage and premature fusion of the synchondroses leading to modifications of foramen magnum shape and size. Partial premature fusion of the coronal sutures and nonossified gaps in frontal bones were also present in *Fgfr3*$^{Y367C/+}$ mice and ACH patients. These data expand the general concept of dwarfism by showing that FGFR3 mutations affect not only the skull base and facial skeleton but also induce anomalies in the skull vault. In conclusion, in ACH and in *Fgfr3*$^{Y367C/+}$ mice not only endochondral ossification but also membranous ossification is affected [20].

## Therapeutic Approaches to Achondroplasia

The first therapeutic approach proposed for the treatment of ACH patients was growth hormone therapy; the effect of this treatment is moderate and the long-term effects remain controversial. Limb lengthening to gain bone length can also be offered to the patients. Such a lengthening process is painful; it takes a long time and may be associated with orthopedic complications.

Potential therapeutic strategies have been emerging for ACH for a few years now. Many nonsurgical strategies aimed at reducing excessive activation of FGFR3 have been proposed as possible treatments to stimulate linear bone growth in ACH. First of all, they include strategies to interfere with FGFR3 synthesis, block its activation, inhibit its tyrosine kinase activity, promote its degradation and antagonize its downstream signals. Many strategies have been borrowed conceptually from the oncological field, which is not surprising because the genetic lesions leading to FGFR3-related skeletal disorders are identical to those found in FGFR3-driven cancers, e.g. bladder tumors and multiple myelomas. Among the therapeutic strategies, we can mention inhibition of FGFR3 tyrosine kinase activity with small molecule tyrosine kinase inhibitors. Two small molecule inhibitors of receptor tyrosine kinase, CHIR-258 and A31, are able to inhibit FGFR3 activation [11, 21]. Therapeutic efficacy of CHIR-258 was demonstrated in a xenograft mouse model of FGFR3 multiple myeloma [21]. A31 was tested in embryonic femur cultures isolated from mutant mice with dwarfism and showed an important correction of the growth defect after 6 days of culture. Two other FGFR3 tyrosine kinase inhibitors, PD173074 and SU5402, inhibit the growth and induce apoptosis of multiple myeloma cells. However, they are not selective for FGFR3. Another approach consists of using monoclonal antibodies to target the extracellular part of the receptor. These studies demonstrated that specific FGFR3 monoclonal antibodies were highly efficient in various bladder cancer cell lines and were able to reduce orthotopic bladder cancer xenograft growth [22]. Today, there are no subsequent reports on the capacity of FGFR3 monoclonal antibodies to stimulate bone growth in vivo [23]. A new therapeutic approach was recently designed with the objective to catch available FGFs using a soluble form of FGFR3. This recombinant soluble FGFR3 therapy was conducted in *Fgfr3*$^{Ach/+}$ mice. The rescue of the bone size and restoration of growth plate maturation were observed in treated *Fgfr3*$^{Ach/+}$ mice. However, additional preclinical studies need to be performed to confirm the viability of this treatment before the initiation of clinical trials [24].

Many signaling molecules and transcription factors are involved during growth plate development and maturation stages. In ACH, the balance between chondrocyte proliferation and differentiation is severely disturbed. Among the factors playing a crucial role, parathyroid hormone (PTH)-related peptide and its receptor (PTHR1) is seen as an important regulator of the proliferation and differentiation of the chondrocytes in the growth plate. In order to correct the proliferation and differentiation defect in ACH, systemic intermittent PTH (1-34) injections were done in *Fgfr3*$^{+/K544E}$ mice. These preclinical studies showed the rescue of the retarded skeletal development [25]. It would be necessary to determine the safety of PTH injection before moving forward to the clinical practice.

Recently, other strategies have emerged and aim at drugs currently used for non-skeletal disorders. The first example is meclozine, an over-the-counter $H_1$-receptor inhibitor used to treat motion sickness. In various cell lines, meclozine was able to promote chondrocyte proliferation and differentiation, and attenuate ERK phosphorylation [26]. In ex vivo culture, the drug increases the longitudinal growth of embryonic normal and *Fgfr3*$^{ach/+}$ tibia explants. Oral administration of meclozine to *Fgfr3*$^{ach/+}$ mice increased longitudinal bone growth but failed to increase the size of the foramen magnum and lumbar spinal canal [27]. In the future, histological analyses of the growth plate need to be performed to confirm the rescue of the growth plate defect. The second example is statin, a cholesterol-lowering drug. Yamashita et al. [28] showed that the addition of statins to culture media rescued the defective chondrogenesis of the ACH-induced pluripotent stem cells and corrected the skeletal development of *Fgfr3*$^{ach/+}$ mice. Today, there is a lot of controversy regarding the use of statins as a therapeutic approach to ACH. Indeed, some papers showed that statin retarded cartilage development and reduced the expression of the principal regulator of the growth plate cartilage [29]. The mechanism by which statin could modify bone growth in ACH needs to be elucidated.

Finally, today, the most promising approach is C-type natriuretic peptide (CNP) for the treatment of ACH. CNP, a 22-amino-acid peptide, and its receptor, natriuretic peptide receptor B (NPR-B), are recognized as important regulators of longitudinal growth. Loss-of-function mutations in *NPR-B* are responsible for acromesomelic dysplasia, Maroteaux type, a disproportionate dwarfism in humans [30]. Mutant mice with a disruption in CNP (Nppc$^{-/-}$) had also disproportionate dwarfism with short limbs [31]. Conversely, skeletal overgrowth has been observed in patients with overexpression of CNP caused by a balanced translocation [32, 33]. The same phenotype was reported in mutant mice [34]. Interestingly, CNP overexpression in the cartilage or continuous delivery of CNP through intravenous infusion normalizes the dwarfism of *Fgfr3*$^{ach/+}$ mice [35, 36], suggesting that CNP is a potential strategy to treat ACH.

The role of the MAPK pathway in mediating FGFR3 activity is illustrated by the dwarfism of mice with constitutive activation of ERK1/MEK1 and conversely by the overgrowth of long bones of mice with ERK1/2 inactivation [37]. The MAPK signaling pathway is regulated by CNP, and CNP and its receptor (NPR-B) inhibit the

FGFR3 downstream MAPK signaling pathway at the level of RAF-1 [18]. However, due to the short half-life of CNP (2 min after intravenous administration) [35, 36], CNP is impracticable as a therapeutic agent as it would require continuous intravenous infusion. To overcome this limitation, the company BioMarin designed and manufactured BMN111, a 39-amino-acid pharmacological variant of CNP. BMN111 mimics the pharmacological activity of native CNP and has an extended half-life due to neutral endopeptidase resistance [18, 38].

The pharmacological activity of BMN111 was tested in vitro using primary human growth plate chondrocytes carrying various *FGFR3* gain-of-function mutations. BMN111 inhibited FGF-mediated ERK1/2 activation in lysates from human primary and immortalized control and mutant chondrocytes carrying the p.Gly380Arg (ACH).

The pharmacological activity of BMN111 was also evaluated ex-vivo using femur explants isolated from *Fgfr3*$^{Y367C/+}$ mice. Co-incubation of the femurs with BMN111 for 6 days led to a significant increase in femur length and correction of the growth plate size and architecture [18].

In vivo experiments were conducted in two *Fgfr3* mouse models. The first experiments were done in *Fgfr3*$^{Ach/+}$ mice. These mutant mice overexpress ACH mutations under the control of the type II collagen promoter. Significant growth was observed in the appendicular and the axial skeletons in treated *Fgfr3*$^{Ach/+}$ mice. An increased size in the growth plate is observed corresponding to a modification in the area of the proliferative and hypertrophic zones [38]. The second mouse model (*Fgfr3*$^{Y367C/+}$) is characterized by a more severe skeletal phenotype than *Fgfr3*$^{Ach/+}$ mice. In this protocol, the *Fgfr3*$^{Y367C/+}$ mice received daily subcutaneous administrations of BMN111 during 20 days. Major phenotypic changes were observed. Significant growth of the tibiae and femurs and an increase in the anterior-posterior diameter of the skull were observed. The BMN111 treatment led to a flattening of the skull with an elongation of the snout, larger paws and digits, and straightening of the tibiae and femurs [18].

The putative hemodynamic effects of BMN111 were tested in cynomolgus monkeys. The study was performed in normal juvenile cynomolgus monkeys. ECG parameters were unaffected at any dose of BMN111, and there were no clinical signs of hypotension or distress at any time during the treatment. An increased growth rate was noted with an enlarged growth plate cartilage area. BMN111 treatment modified the spinal canal at the vertebral lumbar (L2) level [38].

All these promising preclinical data allowed BioMarin to initiate a phase 1 clinical trial in healthy volunteers. The treatment was well tolerated, and a safe dose for the pediatric population was identified. In 2014, 20 years after the identification of the ACH gene, a multinational clinical trial for pediatric patients with ACH has started. One of the objectives is to assess the safety and tolerability of daily administration of BMN111 to children with ACH.

Today, we have entered a new era, and to cure patients with skeletal disorders is not a dream but a way of making dreams become reality.

## References


1 Rousseau F, Bonaventure J, Legeai-Mallet L, Pelet A, Rozet JM, Maroteaux P, Le Merrer M, Munnich A: Mutations in the gene encoding fibroblast growth factor receptor-3 in achondroplasia. Nature 1994;371:252–254.

2 Shiang R, Thompson LM, Zhu YZ, Church DM, Fielder TJ, Bocian M, Winokur ST, Wasmuth JJ: Mutations in the transmembrane domain of FGFR3 cause the most common genetic form of dwarfism, achondroplasia. Cell 1994;78:335–342.

3 Horton WA, Hall JG, Hecht JT: Achondroplasia. Lancet 2007;370:162–172.

4 Baujat G, Legeai-Mallet L, Finidori G, Cormier-Daire V, Le Merrer M: Achondroplasia. Best Pract Res Clin Rheumatol 2008;22:3–18.

5 Krejci P, Prochazkova J, Smutny J, Chlebova K, Lin P, Aklian A, Bryja V, Kozubik A, Wilcox WR: FGFR3 signaling induces a reversible senescence phenotype in chondrocytes similar to oncogene-induced premature senescence. Bone 2010;47:102–110.

6 Gibbs L, Legeai-Mallet L: FGFR3 intracellular mutations induce tyrosine phosphorylation in the Golgi and defective glycosylation. Biochem Biophys Acta 2007;1773:502–512.

7 Legeai-Mallet L, Benoist-Lasselin C, Munnich A, Bonaventure J: Overexpression of FGFR3, Stat1, Stat5 and p21Cip1 correlates with phenotypic severity and defective chondrocyte differentiation in FGFR3-related chondrodysplasias. Bone 2004;34:26–36.

8 Murakami S, Balmes G, McKinney S, Zhang Z, Givol D, de Crombrugghe B: Constitutive activation of MEK1 in chondrocytes causes Stat1-independent achondroplasia-like dwarfism and rescues the Fgfr3-deficient mouse phenotype. Genes Dev 2004;18:290–305.

9 Nowroozi N, Raffioni S, Wang T, Apostol BL, Bradshaw RA, Thompson LM: Sustained ERK1/2 but not STAT1 or 3 activation is required for thanatophoric dysplasia phenotypes in PC12 cells. Hum Mol Genet 2005;14:1529–1538.

10 Delezoide AL, Lasselin-Benoist C, Legeai-Mallet L, Brice P, Senée V, Yayon A, Munnich A, Vekemans M, Bonaventure J: Abnormal FGFR 3 expression in cartilage of thanatophoric dysplasia fetuses. Hum Mol Genet 1997;6:1899–1906.

11 Jonquoy A, Mugniery E, Benoist-Lasselin C, Kaci N, Le Corre L, Barbault F, Girard AL, Le Merrer Y, Busca P, Schibler L, Munnich A, Legeai-Mallet L: A novel tyrosine kinase inhibitor restores chondrocyte differentiation and promotes bone growth in a gain-of-function Fgfr3 mouse model. Hum Mol Genet 2012;21:841–851.

12 Colvin JS, Bohne BA, Harding GW, McEwen DG, Ornitz DM: Skeletal overgrowth and deafness in mice lacking fibroblast growth factor receptor 3. Nat Genet 1996;12:390–397.

13 Deng C, Wynshaw-Boris A, Zhou F, Kuo A, Leder P: Fibroblast growth factor receptor 3 is a negative regulator of bone growth. Cell 1996;84:911–921.

14 Pannier S, Couloigner V, Messaddeq N, Elmaleh-Bergès M, Munnich A, Romand R, Legeai-Mallet L: Activating Fgfr3 Y367C mutation causes hearing loss and inner ear defect in a mouse model of chondrodysplasia. Biochim Biophys Acta 2009;1792:140–147.

15 Chen L, Adar R, Yang X, Monsonego EO, Li C, Hauschka PV, Yayon A, Deng CX: Gly369Cys mutation in mouse FGFR3 causes achondroplasia by affecting both chondrogenesis and osteogenesis. J Clin Invest 1999;104:1517–1525.

16 Wang Y, Spatz MK, Kannan K, Hayk H, Avivi A, Gorivodsky M, Pines M, Yayon A, Lonai P, Givol D: A mouse model for achondroplasia produced by targeting fibroblast growth factor receptor 3. Proc Natl Acad Sci U S A 1999;96:4455–4460.

17 Iwata T, Li CL, Deng CX, Francomano CA: Highly activated Fgfr3 with the K644M mutation causes prolonged survival in severe dwarf mice. Hum Mol Genet 2001;10:1255–1264.

18 Lorget F, Kaci N, Peng J, Benoist-Lasselin C, Mugniery E, Oppeneer T, Wendt DJ, Bell SM, Bullens S, Bunting S, Tsuruda LS, O'Neill CA, Di Rocco F, Munnich A, Legeai-Mallet L: Evaluation of the therapeutic potential of a CNP analog in a Fgfr3 mouse model recapitulating achondroplasia. Am J Hum Genet 2012;91:1108–1114.

19 Reina V, Baujat G, Fauroux B, Couloigner V, Boulanger E, Sainte-Rose C, Maroteaux P, Merrer ML, Cormier-Daire V, Legai-Mallet L, Zerah M, Di Rocco F: Craniovertebral junction anomalies in achondroplastic children. Adv Tech Stand Neurosurg 2014;40:295–312.

20 Mugniery E, Dacquin R, Marty C, Benoist-Lasselin C, de Vernejoul MC, Jurdic P, Munnich A, Geoffroy V, Legeai-Mallet L: An activating Fgfr3 mutation affects trabecular bone formation via a paracrine mechanism during growth. Hum Mol Genet 2012;21:2503–2513.

21 Trudel S, Li ZH, Wei E, Wiesmann M, Chang H, Chen C, Reece D, Heise C, Stewart AK: CHIR-258, a novel, multitargeted tyrosine kinase inhibitor for the potential treatment of t(4;14) multiple myeloma. Blood 2005;105:2941–2948.

22 Gust KM, McConkey DJ, Awrey S, Hegarty PK, Qing J, Bondaruk J, Ashkenazi A, Czerniak B, Dinney CP, Black PC: Fibroblast growth factor receptor 3 is a rational therapeutic target in bladder cancer. Mol Cancer Ther 2013;12:1245–1254.

23 Rauchenberger R, Borges E, Thomassen-Wolf E, Rom E, Adar R, Yaniv Y, Malka M, Chumakov I, Kotzer S, Resnitzky D, Knappik A, Reiffert S, Prassler J, Jury K, Waldherr D, Bauer S, Kretzschmar T, Yayon A, Rothe C: Human combinatorial Fab library yielding specific and functional antibodies against the human fibroblast growth factor receptor 3. J Biol Chem 2003;278:38194–38205.
24 Garcia S, Dirat B, Tognacci T, Rochet N, Mouska X, Bonnafous S, Patouraux S, Tran A, Gual P, Le Marchand-Brustel Y, Gennero I, Gouze E: Postnatal soluble FGFR3 therapy rescues achondroplasia symptoms and restores bone growth in mice. Sci Transl Med 2013;5:203ra124.
25 Xie Y, Su N, Jin M, Qi H, Yang J, Li C, Du X, Luo F, Chen B, Shen Y, Huang H, Xian CJ, Deng C, Chen L: Intermittent PTH (1-34) injection rescues the retarded skeletal development and postnatal lethality of mice mimicking human achondroplasia and thanatophoric dysplasia. Hum Mol Genet 2012;15:3941–3955.
26 Matsushita M, Kitoh H, Ohkawara B, Mishima K, Kaneko H, Ito M, Masuda A, Ishiguro N, Ohno K: Meclozine facilitates proliferation and differentiation of chondrocytes by attenuating abnormally activated FGFR3 signaling in achondroplasia. PLoS One 2013;8:e81569.
27 Matsushita M, Hasegawa S, Kitoh H, Mori K, Ohkawara B, Yasoda A, Masuda A, Ishiguro N, Ohno K: Meclozine promotes longitudinal skeletal growth in transgenic mice with achondroplasia carrying a gain-of-function mutation in the FGFR3 gene. Endocrinology 2015;156:548–554.
28 Yamashita A, Morioka M, Kishi H, Kimura T, Yahara Y, Okada M, Fujita K, Sawai H, Ikegawa S, Tsumaki N: Statin treatment rescues FGFR3 skeletal dysplasia phenotypes. Nature 2014;25:507–511.
29 Bush JR, Bérubé NG, Beier F: A new prescription for growth? Statins, cholesterol and cartilage homeostasis. Osteoarthritis Cartilage 2015;23:503–506.
30 Bartels CF, Bükülmez H, Padayatti P, Rhee DK, van Ravenswaaij-Arts C, Pauli RM, Mundlos S, Chitayat D, Shih LY, Al-Gazali LI, Kant S, Cole T, Morton J, Cormier-Daire V, Faivre L, Lees M, Kirk J, Mortier GR, Leroy J, Zabel B, Kim CA, Crow Y, Braverman NE, van den Akker F, Warman ML: Mutations in the transmembrane natriuretic peptide receptor NPR-B impair skeletal growth and cause acromesomelic dysplasia, type Maroteaux. Am J Hum Genet 2004; 75:27–34.
31 Chusho H, Tamura N, Ogawa Y, Yasoda A, Suda M, Miyazawa T, Nakamura K, Nakao K, Kurihara T, Komatsu Y, Itoh H, Tanaka K, Saito Y, Katsuki M, Nakao K: Dwarfism and early death in mice lacking C-type natriuretic peptide. Proc Natl Acad Sci U S A 2001;98:4016–4021.
32 Bocciardi R, Giorda R, Buttgereit J, Gimelli S, Divizia MT, Beri S, Garofalo S, Tavella S, Lerone M, Zuffardi O, Bader M, Ravazzolo R, Gimelli G: Overexpression of the C-type natriuretic peptide (CNP) is associated with overgrowth and bone anomalies in an individual with balanced t(2;7) translocation. Hum Mutat 2007;28:724–731.
33 Moncla A, Missirian C, Cacciagli P, Balzamo E, Legeai-Mallet L, Jouve JL, Chabrol B, Le Merrer M, Plessis G, Villard L, Philip N: A cluster of translocation breakpoints in 2q37 is associated with overexpression of NPPC in patients with a similar overgrowth phenotype. Hum Mutat 2007;28:1183–1188.
34 Suda M, Ogawa Y, Tanaka K, Tamura N, Yasoda A, Takigawa T, Uehira M, Nishimoto H, Itoh H, Saito Y, Shiota K, Nakao K: Skeletal overgrowth in transgenic mice that overexpress brain natriuretic peptide. Proc Natl Acad Sci U S A 1998;3:2337–2342.
35 Yasoda A, Kitamura H, Fujli T, Kondo E, Murao N, Miura M, Kanamoto N, Komatsu Y, Arai H, Nakao K: A systemic administration of C-type natriuretic peptide as a novel therapeutic strategy for skeletal dysplasias. Endocrinology 2009;150:3138–3144.
36 Yasoda A, Kamatsu Y, Chuscho H, Miyazama T, Ozasa A, Miura M, Kurihara T, Rogi T, Tanaka S, Suda M, Tamura N, Ogawa Y, Nakao K: Overexpression of CNP in chondrocytes rescues achondroplasia through a MAPK-dependent pathway. Nat Med 2004;10:80–86.
37 Sebastian A, Matsushita T, Kawanami A, Mackem S, Landreth GE, Murakami S: Genetic inactivation of ERK1 and ERK2 in chondrocytes promotes bone growth and enlarges the spinal canal. J Orthop Res 2011;29:375–379.
38 Wendt DJ, Dvorak-Ewell M, Bullens S, Lorget F, Bell SM, Peng J, Castillo S, Aoyagi-Scharber M, O'Neill CA, Krejci P, Wilcox WR, Rimoin DL, Bunting S: Neutral endopeptidase-resistant C-type natriuretic peptide variant represents a new therapeutic approach for treatment of fibroblast growth factor receptor 3-related dwarfism. J Pharmacol Exp Ther 2015;353:132–149.

Laurence Legeai-Mallet, PhD
INSERM U1163, Institut Imagine
Université Paris Descartes-Sorbonne Paris Cité
24, Boulevard du Montparnasse, FR–75015 Paris (France)
E-Mail laurence.legeai-mallet@inserm.fr

Cappa M, Cianfarani S, Ghizzoni L, Loche S, Maghnie M (eds): Advanced Therapies in Pediatric Endocrinology and Diabetology. Endocr Dev. Basel, Karger, 2016, vol 30, pp 106–129 (DOI: 10.1159/000439337)

# Therapeutic Neuroendocrine Agonist and Antagonist Analogs of Hypothalamic Neuropeptides as Modulators of the Hypothalamic-Pituitary-Gonadal Axis

Claire L. Newton[a, c] • Ross C. Anderson[a, c] • Robert P. Millar[a–c]

[a]Centre for Neuroendocrinology, Department of Immunology, Faculty of Health Sciences, and [b]The Mammal Research Institute, Department of Zoology and Entomology, Faculty of Natural and Agricultural Sciences, University of Pretoria, Pretoria, and [c]UCT/MRC Receptor Biology Unit, Medical Biochemistry and Institute of Infectious Diseases and Molecular Medicine, University of Cape Town, Cape Town, South Africa

**Abstract**

Reproductive hormones play a role at all stages of life and affect most tissues of the body. Gonadotropin-releasing hormone (GnRH) synthesized in the hypothalamus stimulates the secretion of gonadotropins which in turn stimulate gonadal sex hormone production and gamete formation. This hypothalamic-pituitary-gonadal (HPG) axis has, therefore, been the target for the development of numerous drugs which regulate it at various points. These include sex steroid agonists and antagonists, inhibitors of sex steroid biosynthesis, and GnRH agonists and antagonists, which have found extensive applications in treating numerous conditions such as precocious puberty, delayed puberty, prostate cancer, benign prostatic hyperplasia, endometriosis, uterine fibroids and also in in vitro fertilization protocols. The novel neuroendocrine peptides, kisspeptin (KP) and neurokinin B (NKB), were recently discovered as upstream regulators of GnRH, and inactivating mutations of KP and NKB ligands or receptors result in a failure to progress through puberty. Agonists and antagonists of KP and NKB are being developed as more subtle modulators of the HPG axis. These new drugs offer additional and alternative therapeutic options in pediatric and adult hormone-dependent diseases.



The development of synthetic molecules that modulate reproductive hormones has had a major impact on human lifestyle and health. The contraceptive pill for women is considered to be amongst the most important contributions to women's liberation and increased participation in professional and public life. On the other hand, anabolic steroids are the most commonly utilized enhancers of competitive athletic per-

**Table 1.** Applications of HPG axis hormone analogs

| |
|---|
| Gonadal function |
| Female and male contraception |
| Female and male infertility – induction of ovulation/IVF |
| Delayed puberty |
| Precocious puberty |
| Hypothalamic amenorrhea |
| Sex steroid-dependent reproductive diseases |
| Prostate cancer |
| Benign prostatic hyperplasia |
| Endometriosis |
| Uterine fibroids |
| PCOS |
| Breast cancer |
| Ovarian cancer |
| Muscle and bone |
| Bone loss (osteoporosis) |
| Muscle loss in aging and catabolic states |
| Brain |
| Cognitive function |
| Senile dementia and Alzheimer's disease |
| Metabolism |
| Obesity |
| Hypogonadism in diabetes mellitus |
| Reduced lean body mass in aging |

formance, while estrogen and androgen antagonists, and inhibitors of their synthesis and bioconversion, are extensively employed as therapeutics for two of the most prevalent cancers in men and women: breast and prostatic cancers. A wide range of tissues are stimulated by sex steroid hormones, and a number of hormone-dependent diseases arise from dysfunctional sex hormone stimulation including delayed puberty, precocious puberty, benign prostatic hyperplasia, prostatic cancer, ovarian cancer, polycystic ovary syndrome (PCOS), endometriosis, uterine fibroids, muscle wasting, metabolism and cognitive function (table 1).

Diverse external and internal inputs such as photoperiod, metabolic products and nutrients, growth factors, stress, infection and inflammation, as well as many central and peripheral growth factors and hormones regulate the reproductive system. These inputs are integrated in the brain and hypothalamus to regulate the biosynthesis and secretion of gonadotropin-releasing hormone (GnRH; fig. 1). GnRH is conducted by portal vessels to the anterior pituitary where it binds to the GnRH receptor (GnRHR) on gonadotropes to recruit intracellular signaling machinery which stimulates the biosynthesis and secretion of the gonadotropins, luteinizing hormone (LH) and follicle-stimulating hormone (FSH) [1, 2]. LH and FSH then stimulate the ovaries and testes to produce gametes and steroid and peptide hormones. These hormones give feedback in positive and negative modalities at the hypothalamus and pituitary to regulate the reproductive hormone cascade (fig. 1).

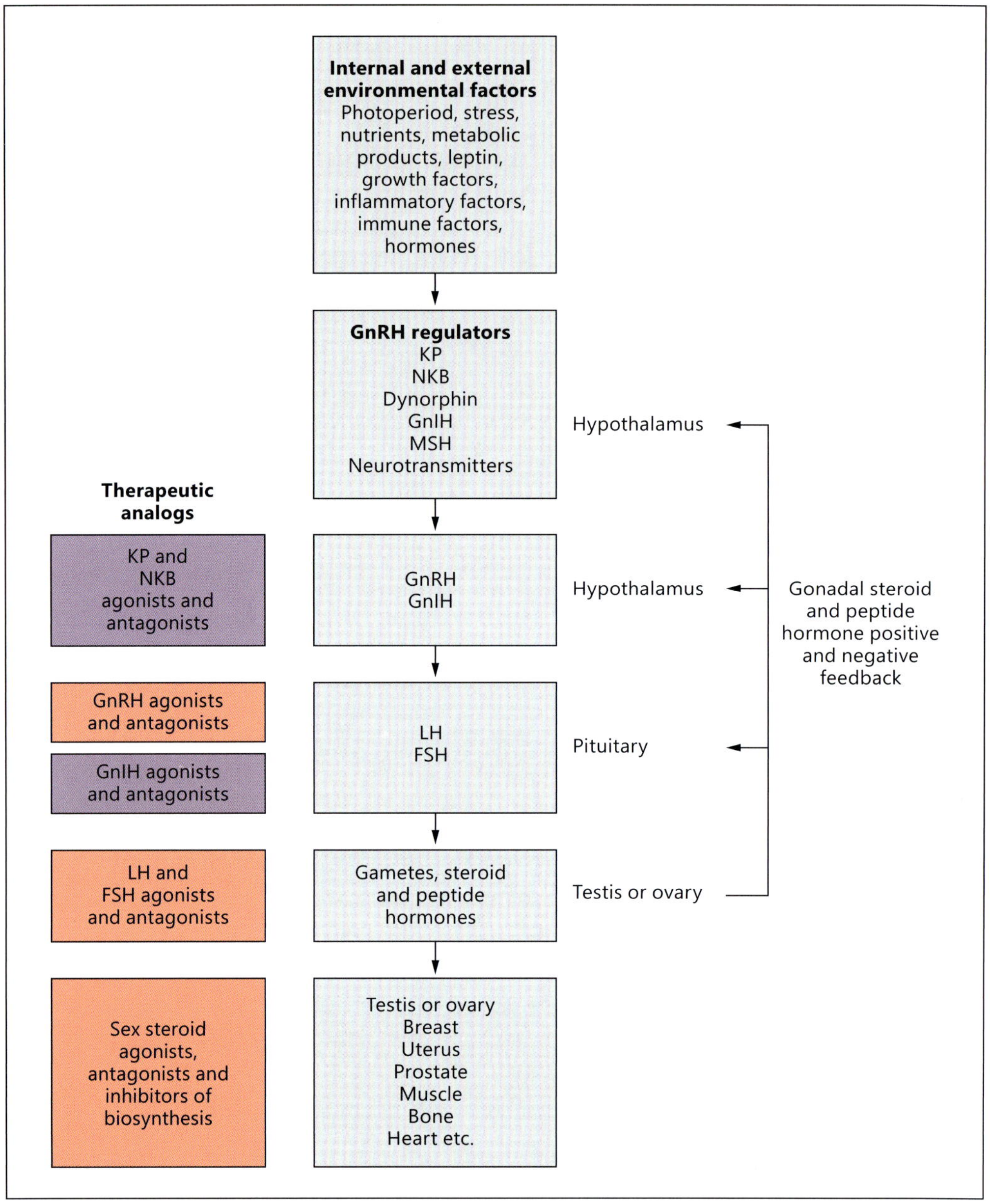


**Fig. 1.** The reproductive hormone cascade and therapeutic analogs that target the cascade. The figure shows the diverse internal and external factors regulating brain neuroendocrine neuropeptides, which in turn regulate downstream GnRH, pituitary gonadotropins and gonadal hormones. Positive and negative feedback by gonadal steroids and peptides is also shown. Analogs have been developed that target all levels of the cascade. Those in clinical use are highlighted in red boxes, and those in purple boxes are being developed but are not yet in clinical use. MSH = Melanocyte-stimulating hormone. Reproduced from Millar and Newton [8].

The array of external and internal factors regulating GnRH do so through a complex neuronal network in the central nervous system (CNS) and hypothalamus which secrete neurotransmitters and neuropeptides which regulate the GnRH neuron. Inactivating mutations in kisspeptin (KP) and neurokinin B (NKB) or their cognate receptors recently highlighted the crucial role of these neuropeptides in GnRH neuron activation, as these mutations result in a failure to progress through puberty and ensuing adult infertility [3–8]. Mutations in these neuropeptide receptors can also result in constitutive activity resulting in precocious puberty.

All of the hormones in the cascade from the brain to the pituitary, gonads and peripheral tissues are targets for the development of analogs which ultimately modulate the production of gametes and the sex steroid hormones which impact on most tissues of the body. The sites of current and potential intervention in the reproductive hormone cascade are indicated in figure 1.

Sex steroid agonists, antagonists and inhibitors of their synthesis have been extensively employed for contraception and hormone-dependent diseases for many years. GnRH and its analogs have likewise been extensively employed in treating hormone-dependent diseases. Natural and recombinant gonadotropins are the mainstay of the treatment of delayed puberty, infertility and assisted reproductive technologies such as in vitro fertilization (IVF). Although the novel neuropeptides KP, NKB and gonadotropin-inhibitory hormone (GnIH/RFRP3), which regulate GnRH neurons, are potential targets for regulating the reproductive system, the use of agonist and antagonist analogs has currently been largely restricted to animal studies but show promise as regulators of the reproductive system in humans.

This chapter, which has drawn extensively on previous reviews by us, describes the physiology, development and application of analogs of GnRH, KP and NKB [1, 2, 8]. The reader is referred to Millar and Newton [8] for a comprehensive list of references due to the restricted number in this review.

## Gonadotropin-Releasing Hormone Analogs

### *Background*

As the central initiator of the reproductive hormonal cascade, GnRH was first isolated from mammalian hypothalami as the decapeptide (pGlu-His-Trp-Ser-Tyr-Gly-Leu-Arg-Pro-Gly-$NH_2$) [1, 2, 8]. GnRH is synthesized from a precursor polypeptide by enzymatic processing and packaged in storage granules that are transported down axons to the median eminence from where it is released in synchronized pulses into the hypophyseal portal system every 30–120 min to stimulate gonadotrope biosynthesis and secretion of LH and FSH. Each GnRH pulse stimulates a pulse of LH, but FSH pulses are less clear in view of its longer half-life. In the female, the frequency of pulses is highest at the LH surge of ovulation and lowest during the luteal phase of the ovarian cycle. The asynchronous patterns of LH and FSH release which is crucial for the cycle result from changes in GnRH pulse frequency, modulating effects of gonadal steroid and peptide hormones on FSH and LH responses to GnRH, and differences in the half-lives of the two hormones. High-frequency pulses favor LH secretion while low frequency favors FSH secretion. In addition, LH is stored in secretory granules and is dependent on GnRH for secretion, while FSH is constitutively secreted and is therefore more dependent on biosynthesis.

### *Natural Gonadotropin-Releasing Hormone and Peptide Agonists and Antagonists*

The primary structure of GnRH determined in mammals was initially thought to be conserved throughout vertebrates. However, the demonstration that amphibian, bird, fish and reptile GnRHs had different charge properties [9] led to the structural elucidation of a novel form in chickens [10] and subsequently to a variety of structures in vertebrates and invertebrates [11]. These structural variants represent 'experiments of nature' over many million years of evolution and provide insight into functionally important residues, which revealed that the amino COOH- and $NH_2$-terminal domains are highly conserved, indicating that they are important for receptor binding and activation. $Gly^6$ is also highly conserved in vertebrates to facilitate folding of the peptide. The amino acid in position eight is highly variable across species, and $Arg^8$ in mammalian GnRH is essential for high-affinity binding to mammalian receptors through interaction with an acidic residue in extracellular loop three.

Physicochemical studies have indicated that mammalian GnRH takes up a folded conformation around $Gly^6$ wherein $NH_2$ and COOH termini are closely apposed, allowing these conserved domains to bind and activate the receptor (fig. 2). The achiral $Gly^6$ (absence of a side chain) facilitates the formation of a β-II′-type turn. When $Gly^6$ is substituted with a D-amino acid, the β-II′ conformation is enhanced and binding affinity is increased 10- to 100-fold [1, 2, 12]. This substitution is, therefore, utilized in all GnRH agonist and antagonist analogs. The substitution has the added advantage of conveying resistance to proteolytic enzyme cleavage. Substitution of the $NH_2$-terminal amino acids (which are involved in receptor activation) with D-amino acids which have large hydrophobic side chains (e.g. D-tryptophan, D-phenylalanine, D-naphthylalanine and other unnatural D-amino acids) produces antagonists (fig. 2). These substitutions also result in binding to plasma proteins such as albumin, thus further enhancing half-life in the circulation [1, 2, 12]. Substitution of the carboxyl-terminal Gly-$NH_2$ with alkyl moieties (e.g. ethylamide) conveys further resistance to proteolysis without compromising binding affinity [1, 2, 12]. These elements form the basis of all GnRH analogs which are currently used in therapies (fig. 3).

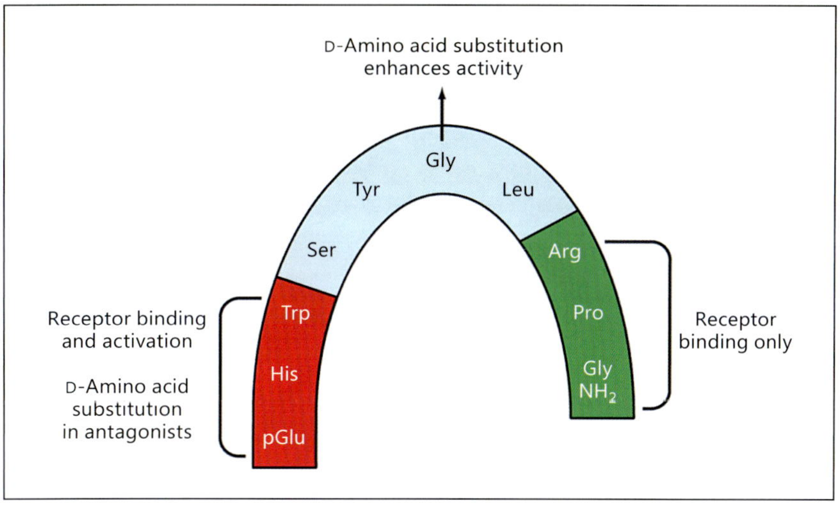


**Fig. 2.** Schematic representation of mammalian GnRH in the folded conformation, in which it is bound to the GnRH receptor in gonadotropes. The molecule is bent around the achiral glycine in position 6. Substitution with D-amino acids in this position stabilizes the folded conformation, increases binding affinity and decreases metabolic clearance. This feature is incorporated in all agonist and antagonist analogs. The amino (red) and carboxyl (green) termini are involved in receptor binding. The amino terminus alone is involved in receptor activation and substitutions in this region produce antagonists. Adapted from Millar and Newton [8].

### *Steroid-Gonadotropin-Releasing Hormone Bifunctional Conjugates*

Although GnRH analogs are the mainstay of prostatic cancer treatment, the total ablation of androgen results in side effects such as hot flushes, loss of libido and bone loss. To counteract these deleterious side effects, we contemplated conjugating estrogen to a GnRH antagonist. We first demonstrated proof of principle by attaching progesterone by an ester linkage to D-Lys in position 6 of the GnRH antagonist. The conjugate molecule retained full GnRH antagonist activity in vitro and in vivo in marmosets as well as high progestogenic activity [13]. We previously produced estrogen-GnRH analog conjugates (fig. 4) and are currently investigating the properties of these molecules as inhibitors of prostatic cancer and maintenance of bone density, libido and prevention of hot flushes.

### *Small-Molecule Nonpeptide Orally Active Gonadotropin-Releasing Hormone Antagonists*

Pharmaceutical companies and a number of small biotech companies have pursued the development of nonpeptide orally bioavailable GnRH antagonists in order to overcome the requirement of injection of peptide analogs. Orally active molecules provide

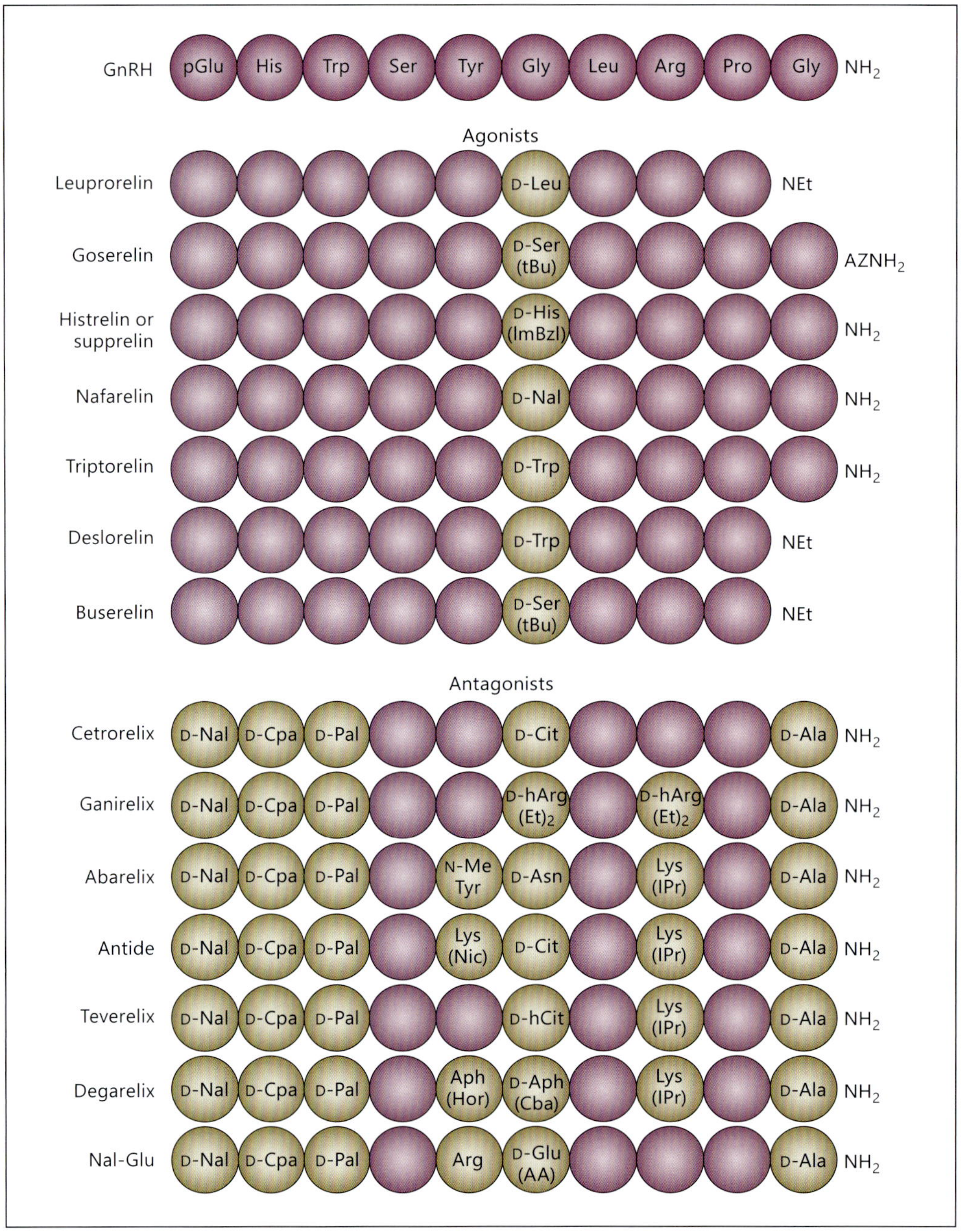


**Fig. 3.** GnRH agonist and antagonist peptide analogs in clinical practice or in clinical development. The mammalian GnRH sequence is shown above in purple circles and substitutions are shown in brown circles. All analogs have a D-amino acid substitution in position 6 to enhance the folding of the molecule and increase binding affinity and decrease degradation. Carboxyl-terminal substitutions further decrease degradation. All antagonists have substitutions in the amino-terminal domain, which ablates receptor activation. Permission to adapt from Millar et al. [1] was obtained from the Endocrine Society.

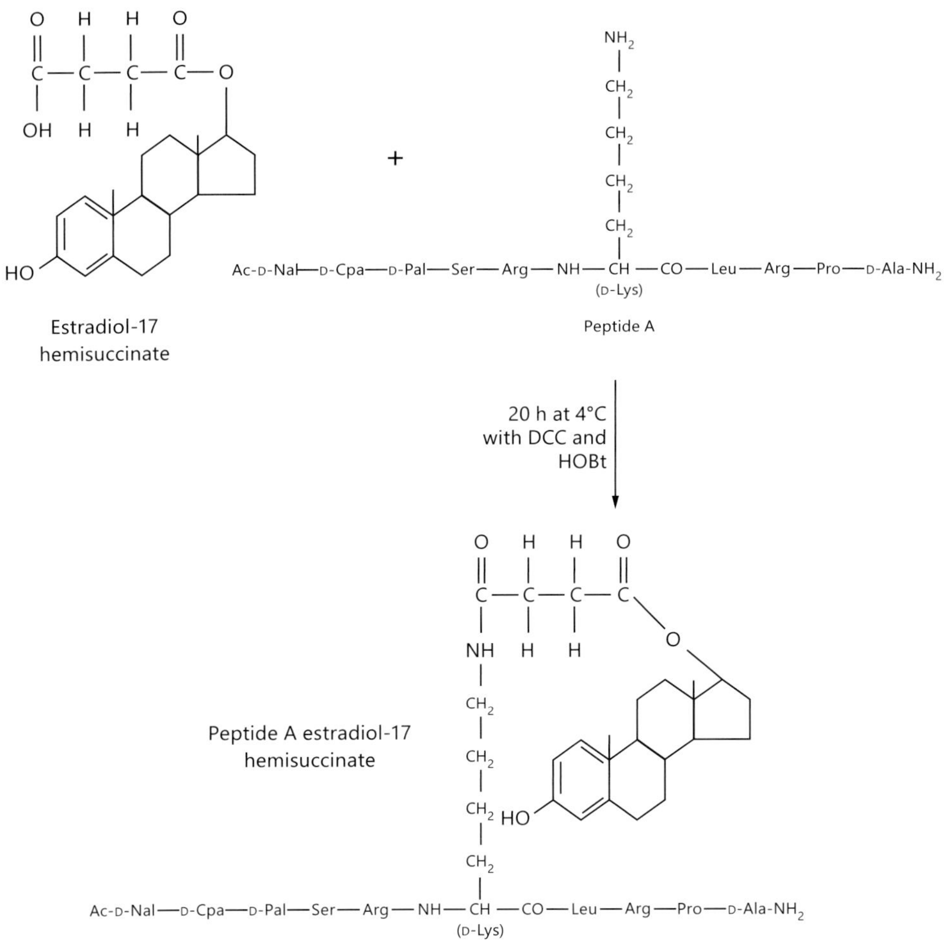


**Fig. 4.** Synthesis of GnRH antagonist conjugate with estradiol. Estradiol hemisuccinate is conjugated to D-lysine in position six of the antagonist using N,N′-dicyclohexyl-carbodiimide (DCC) and hydroxybenzotriazole (HOBt). The conjugate retains full antagonist activity and high estrogenic activity.

the potential for titrating dose to accomplish partial inhibition of sex steroid hormones which is difficult with injectable peptide antagonists. These may have value in partial inhibition of sex steroids in precocious puberty. Partial inhibition is also desirable in certain hormone-dependent diseases such as endometriosis and benign prostatic hyperplasia to ameliorate the pathology without inducing the unwanted side effects of loss of libido and bone, and hot flushes associated with total gonadal steroid inhibition using GnRH analogs. Fourteen chemical classes of compounds have been developed [8]. Of the very large spectrum of analogs which have been developed, only compounds from Neurocrine Biosciences and Takeda have entered the clinic. The compounds exhibit high receptor binding affinity and good bioavailability, and pharmacokinetic and pharmacodynamic profiles. Neurocrine Biosciences have demonstrated good dose-response relations for elagolix, which allows dosing for partial LH and steroid suppression. The primary therapeutic target is currently endometriosis, and elagolix is in phase 2 for this indication. There is also potential application in partial androgen suppression in benign prostatic hyperplasia and precocious puberty. It appears that the binding sites of the nonpeptide GnRH antagonists overlap with the orthosteric binding site of GnRH [8]. Although a number of small-molecule GnRH antagonists have been developed, to date nonpeptide agonists have not been described.

Loss-of-function mutations in the GnRHR have been reported in patients suffering from hypogonadotropic hypogonadism [1]. The majority of these result from misfolding of the receptor and a failure to traffic to the cell surface. Cell-permeant small-molecule GnRH analogs are able to penetrate into the cell and stabilize the mutant GnRHR, thereby acting as 'pharmacoperones' which 'rescue' cell surface expression of intracellularly retained mutant GnRHRs [see ref. 14 for a comprehensive review].

## Gonadotropin-Releasing Hormone Receptor-Gonadotropin-Releasing Hormone Interactions

The GnRHR was first cloned from a gonadotrope cell line [15] and subsequently from many vertebrate and invertebrate species [1]. The receptor is a G protein-coupled receptor (GPR) with seven characteristic transmembrane domains connected by extracellular and intracellular loop domains. Uniquely, there is an absence of a carboxyl-terminal tail which is responsible for rapid (minutes) ligand-induced desensitization of GPRs. Thus, the GnRHR is not rapidly desensitized, probably to facilitate prolonged LH secretion which is necessary for ovulation. Nevertheless, prolonged exposure (1–3 weeks) to GnRH agonists induces a decline in circulating gonadotropin and sex steroids in humans. This is a pharmacological phenomenon, as opposed to rapid desensitization in other GPRs which is designed to terminate signaling. The application of long-term desensitization utilizing GnRH agonists is described below.

Information on the three-dimensional structure of the GnRHR is essential for a complete understanding of its molecular functioning and binding to GnRH. GnRHR molecular models based on the crystal structures of the other GPRs have been valuable in analog development [1, 16].

### *Therapeutic Applications of Gonadotropin-Releasing Hormone and Gonadotropin-Releasing Hormone Analogs*

Pulsatile delivery of 100 μg of natural GnRH every hour (simulating hypothalamic release) has been successfully used to stimulate fertility in hypothalamic hypogonadism resulting from congenital conditions such as Kallman's syndrome and nutritional conditions such as anorexia nervosa, obesity and diabetes mellitus. This treatment modality is also effective in stimulating testis descent in cryptorchism and delayed puberty.

However, the major applications are in the use of GnRH agonists (through gonadotrope desensitization) and GnRH antagonists to inhibit gonadotropin and sex steroid secretion for the treatment of hormone-dependent diseases and in IVF to prevent ovulation and facilitate successful oocyte retrieval (table 1). GnRH agonists (e.g. triptorelin and leuprolide) are formulated as slow-release depot preparations in biodegradable polymers. When injected intramuscularly (about 3–5 mg), these preparations release approximately 100 μg per day for 1 month. Some preparations (e.g. histrelin) are capable of suppressing gonadotropin for 12 months. The disadvantage of GnRH agonists is the initial stimulation of gonadotropin and sex steroids for the first 1–2 weeks prior to the onset of desensitization. This feature results in the 'flare' of the condition in hormone-dependent diseases. This can be managed by concurrent administration of inhibitors of steroid biosynthesis or steroid receptor antagonists. A further disadvantage is that desensitization with agonists requires a longer treatment period when used for the induction of follicle development for oocyte retrieval in IVF. Thus agonists are being increasingly replaced with antagonists as they do not induce disease flare as there is an immediate inhibition of gonadotropin and sex steroids, with a brief delay corresponding to the half-life of the hormones. The first GnRH antagonists developed produced an undesirable histaminic reaction. This was due to a basic-x-basic amino acid motif, and current antagonists avoid this structural feature and are free of histaminic activity. Although GnRH antagonists avoid the flare phenomenon, the significant disadvantage of peptide GnRH antagonists when compared with agonists is that much higher doses are required to continually compete with endogenous GnRH which increases as a result of the decline in sex steroids and concomitant removal of negative feedback on GnRH secretion. Consequently, monthly depot preparations of GnRH antagonist contain about 100 mg or more in contrast to monthly preparations of 3–5 mg GnRH agonists.

The mechanism of GnRH agonist desensitization is widely regarded as being through GnRH receptor 'down-regulation'. This is an oxymoron as the actions of the agonists would be nullified if there was a decline of GnRH receptors on which to act. The multiple mechanisms of desensitization cannot be enumerated here. Suffice to say that the gonadotrope continues to respond to GnRH agonist but fails to elaborate and secrete biologically active gonadotropins. Although circulating α gonadotropin subunit is elevated in patients on long-term GnRH agonist treatment, the biologically active α/β gonadotropin heterodimers are very low, thus down-regulation of gonadal activity is predominantly due to altered biosynthesis [17].

GnRH analog application in prostatic cancer is by far the greatest and is the preferred treatment for this condition. There is increased survival and a reduction in prostate-specific antigen and pain. GnRH analogs are also employed in almost all cycles for IVF treatment to avoid the spontaneous LH surge and loss of oocytes before laparoscopic retrieval. Other applications of GnRH analogs include endometriosis, which has a prevalence of 6–10% in women and 20–40% in infertile women. Improvement of pain is reported in 75% of women on GnRH analog therapy, but there appears to be no improvement in pregnancy rates. GnRH analog therapy has been reported to be beneficial in PCOS (the most common endocrine disorder in women), uterine fibroids (the most common solid tumor in women) and dysfunctional uterine bleeding.

GnRH analogs in combination with anti-estrogen were more effective than either treatment alone in premenopausal women with metastatic estrogen-positive breast cancer. Ovarian and endometrial cancers apparently express GnRH and GnRHR, and there are indications of direct cell cycle arrest and efficacy in clinical trials [16]. A number of studies have utilized GnRH analogs to inhibit gonadal activity in an attempt to protect the gonads prior to cytotoxic chemotherapy, but the effectiveness is still uncertain. The treatment has been widely employed in pediatric oncology in an attempt to preserve fertility.

The objective of GnRH analog therapy in hormone-dependent diseases is to lower sex steroid hormones. However, this gives rise to unwanted side effects in prolonged treatment, such as hot flushes, vaginal dryness, irregular vaginal bleeding, loss of libido, decreased lean body mass and bone loss. These symptoms may be alleviated by intermittent treatment with GnRH analogs or by 'add-back' therapy of appropriate sex steroids (e.g. estrogen in men being treated for prostatic cancer who experience hot flushes, lowered libido and bone loss). A novel approach is the development and use of conjugates of GnRH analogs and sex steroids in which a D-Lys in position six is conjugated to the appropriate sex steroid (fig. 4). These conjugates retain full GnRH analog and steroid activity within a single molecule [13].

In children with precocious puberty, GnRH agonists are very effective in halting the advance through puberty and holding it in check until the patient reaches an appropriate age at which stage treatment is withdrawn and the adolescent can proceed through puberty. Interestingly, there is little consideration of potential deleterious effects of long-term castrate levels of sex hormones. Serious thought should be given to low-dose replacement of sex steroids or treatment with GnRH-steroid conjugates, or titrating sex steroid suppression with orally active GnRH antagonists such as elagolix, or with KP and NKB antagonists, which do not suppress sex steroids to the same extent.

A perceived potential disadvantage of GnRH peptide analogs is the requirement to administer by injection as they are proteolytically cleaved in the digestive tract and not orally bioavailable. However, the need for frequent injection has been overcome by formulating slow-release depot preparations which ensure patient compliance such as in precocious puberty. Indeed many patients prefer this mode of administration. Furthermore, unlike orally active small-molecule drugs, they are modified versions of the natural hormone and thus have potentially fewer off-target side effects.

## Kisspeptin Analogs

### *Background*

Although the GnRH neuron is the final neuroendocrine conduit for the influence of diverse internal and external factors regulating reproduction, the absence of receptors for these inputs on GnRH neurons presented a conundrum. In particular sex steroid hormone receptors which are required for negative and positive feedback by steroids on GnRH secretion are largely absent from GnRH neurons.

This suggested the existence of steroid-responsive neurons which regulate GnRH neurons. The breakthrough in identifying such neurons came with the observation that inactivating mutations in genes encoding the human and mouse KP receptors *(GPR54/Gpr54)* resulted in a failure to progress through puberty [5, 6]. An inactivating mutation in the human *KiSS-1* gene encoding KP also resulted in a failure to achieve puberty [3], thus confirming KP and GPR54 as cognate ligand and receptor partners.

The discovery that the KPs and their cognate receptor GPR54 play a key neuroendocrine role in the regulation of reproduction [3, 5, 6] is regarded as a milestone of equivalent importance to the discovery of GnRH more than three decades earlier. The KPs are members of a group of peptides known as RF-amides characterized by an Arg-Phe-$NH_2$ motif at the COOH terminus. RF-amides signal through GPRs which are involved in numerous physiological and pathophysiological processes, including control of food intake, pain, inflammatory responses, development and metabolism. The *KiSS-1* gene translates into a 145-amino-acid secretory polypeptide with a signal sequence followed by a 119-amino-acid sequence which is processed to a 54-amino-acid peptide (KP-54) in man. The 54-amino-acid peptide is further proteolytically processed to COOH-terminal peptides of 14, 13 and 10 amino acids, all of which are biologically active [18]. The 10-amino-acid peptide (KP-10) has full intrinsic biological activity. However, the 54-amino-acid peptide has a longer half-life and therefore increased LH-releasing activity than the shorter forms in vivo.

KP-10 potently stimulates LH, FSH and gonadal steroid secretion when administered both centrally and systemically [8]. KP stimulation of gonadotropins is ablated by co-administration of GnRH antagonist, thus demonstrating that KP acts through the stimulation of GnRH secretion. Moreover, GnRH neurons express GPR54 and KP stimulates GnRH secretion. Intravenous infusion of KP-54 in normal men increases circulating LH and FSH. Acute intravenous administration of KP-10 has similar stimulatory effects on gonadotropin secretion in men over a dose range of 0.01–1 μg/kg [19]. The stimulatory effect of KP administration to normal women is greatest during the preovulatory phase of the menstrual cycle [20].

Significantly, KP neurons express steroid hormone receptors, and gonadectomy in rodents increases detectable KP cell numbers and mRNA expression levels in the arcuate nucleus (ARC), and steroid replacement reverses this. While KP neurons in the ARC mediate steroid negative feedback control on GnRH neurons, another population in rodents in the anterior ventral paraventricular nucleus mediates the estrogen positive feedback of the ovulatory LH surge. This anatomically linked functional dimorphism of KP neurons is not evident in sheep, monkeys and humans as both types of neurons (regulated positively and negatively by estrogen) appear to be localized in the ARC.

In order to ensure survival of offspring, reproduction is finely tuned to the availability of nutrients and metabolic status. KP appears to have a major mediating role in the dialogue between nutrition and metabolism with reproduction. This relationship is of particular significance in the context of the rising global prevalence of infertility, obesity and secondary pathologies such as diabetes. Substantial data support a central role for the KP/GPR54 system in mediating the effects of metabolism on the reproductive system. A link between leptin secretion from adipose tissue and KP gene expression is suggested by the observation that *KiSS-1* expression in the ARC is reduced in castrated leptin-deficient ob/ob mice and is increased by administration of leptin. In addition, streptozotocin-induced diabetes mellitus results in reduced *KiSS-1* mRNA expression and gonadotropin secretion. Fasting reduces *KiSS-1* mRNA expression in the rat hypothalamus, and KP administration reverses starvation-induced hypogonadotropism, with GPR54 mRNA expression similarly affected. Metabolic effects on reproduction in humans which appear to involve KP dysregulation include hypothalamic amenorrhea (anorexia nervosa being an extreme example) and PCOS, which is characterized by increased LH pulse frequency and is often associated with obesity. For detailed references to the diverse physiological and pathophysiological regulation of KP, the reader is referred to comprehensive reviews [18, 21, 22].

In the majority of studies on the physiological and pathophysiological regulation of KP, the end point measures were KP mRNA and/or KP peptide in tissue. There is therefore no direct evidence that these manipulations alter the *secretion* of KP. An exception is the single study demonstrating that KP antiserum inhibits the ovulatory LH surge, implying that increased KP secretion elicits the LH surge. In order to directly elucidate the role of KP secretion and GPR54 activation in physiological processes, the development of KP antagonists is an essential tool.

An understanding of the structure of KP is valuable in this endeavor. KP-54 and the smaller processed peptides of 14, 13 and 10 amino acids in length have been shown to bind to and activate the receptor with equal potency. The minimal10-amino-acid sequence of the COOH terminus has been used to design KP agonists and antagonists. The activation domain is interpreted to reside within the 5 most amino-terminal residues which is dominated by hydrophobic residues while the binding domain resides predominantly within the 5 most carboxyl-terminal residues which contains both hydrophobic and charged residues.

Two approaches were employed in the development of peptide analogs. In alanine scanning, each residue is systematically substituted with alanine which lacks a functional side chain, thus revealing whether the side chain is of importance or not. Using this approach, two groups revealed that alanine substitutions for $Phe^6$ and $Phe^{10}$ of

KP-10 significantly reduced binding and activation of GPR54 in vitro and in vivo, indicating that their side chain groups are critical to peptide activity [23]. Substitution of $Arg^9$ with alanine also significantly decreased binding and activation as did substitutions of $Leu^8$. Thus, $Phe^6$, $Arg^9$ and $Phe^{10}$ constitute a binding pharmacophore with proposed stacking of phenyl rings of $Phe^6$ and $Phe^{10}$ flanked by $Arg^9$ and $Leu^8$ with side chains orientated on the opposite side of the peptide. The second approach involves amino acid substitutions based on the knowledge of the KP-10 structure. This involves making either conservative changes at positions of interest, such as changing the side chain but not the overall charge of a residue, or changing L-amino acids to D-amino acids to assess the positioning of side chains. Radical structural changes can also be made to change the charge or flexibility of the analog.

### *Kisspeptin Agonists*

Systematic natural and unnatural amino acid substitution was used in the development of KP peptide agonists to target cancers and hormone-dependent diseases [24, 25]. These studies and data in patients confirmed that the critical pharmacophore of $Phe^6$, $Arg^9$ and $Phe^{10}$ must be retained or altered with conservative amino acid substitutions. Other positions in the KP-10 amino acid sequence were subject to a range of substitutions to provide resistance to degradation and improve pharmacokinetics. A series of potent agonists at GPR54 were produced [24, 25].

Two of these agonists at GPR54 (KiSS1-305 and TAK-448) were studied in rats for short-term gonadotropin and steroid hormone stimulation and long-term inhibition through desensitization [26]. With both analogs, testosterone was reduced to castration levels within 3 days and remained depleted throughout the 30-day treatment period. The mechanism of desensitization seemed to be predominantly at the level of the GnRH neuron. Remarkably, the suppression of testosterone levels was apparently more pronounced and faster, and reproductive organ weights were more reduced, than after administration of the GnRH analog leuprorelin. This result is unexpected, as KP stimulation of LH in humans and animals is much less than that of GnRH, and KP antagonists only partially suppress LH, which suggests that a KP-independent component of GnRH secretion exists. Thus, effects of desensitization with KP agonists would be expected to be less effective than that of GnRH agonists.

### *Kisspeptin Antagonists*

Truncation of KP to the last 5 amino acids results in retention of some binding but ablated signaling capacity [23]. Substitutions in this pentapeptide failed to improve binding and further exploration was abandoned in favor of making substitutions in the full-length KP-10. During the course of systematic substitution

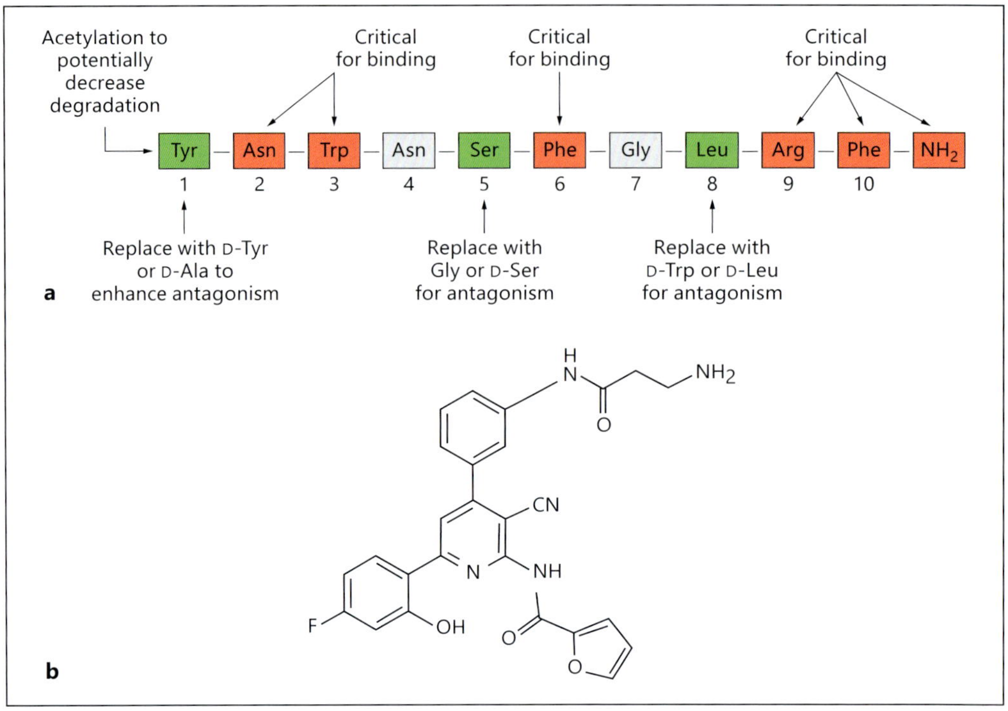


**Fig. 5. a** Consensus structure of KP antagonists. Residues that are important for receptor binding and retained in analogs are shown in red and residues involved in receptor activation, and thus are substituted in antagonists, are shown in green. Residues shown in grey could be substituted without major effects. The substitution of serine at position 5 with glycine allowed flexibility and greater tolerance of the substitutions required for antagonist activity. **b** Nonpeptide small-molecule KP antagonist 15a, which shows high binding affinity for GPR54 and antagonism of KP in vitro and in vivo. Reproduced from Millar and Newton [8].

of each of the 10 amino acids, a consensus sequence emerged for analogs which retained binding but did not recruit signaling. They antagonized KP-10 stimulation of signaling in cells expressing the human GPR54. This is summarized in figure 5a.

The most valuable additional substitution for antagonism was the replacement of $Leu^8$ with D-Trp. This peptide (210) exhibited high binding affinity (7.3 nM) and inhibition of 10 nM KP-10 stimulation of inositol phosphate generation. This peptide was acetylated at the amino terminus in an attempt to reduce degradation and was effective in inhibiting LH in animal models [23]. Another advance was the substitution of $Tyr^1$ with acetylated D-Ala to produce peptide 234, which was a potent antagonist in a wide range of ex vivo and in vivo animal studies [23].

A penetratin sequence was also added to the amino terminus of 234 to create a peptide capable of penetrating the blood-brain barrier (peptide 271). Again, this antagonist was active in vivo and it may be a valuable tool with which to compare the effects of 234 and tease out potential differences in activities at GnRH nerve terminals (234) as opposed to both terminals and cell bodies (271).

*Small-Molecule Antagonists*

Small-molecule nonpeptide KP antagonists derived from a 2-acylamino-4,6-diphenylpyridine scaffold have been developed. Kobayashi et al. [27] adopted a combinatorial chemistry approach to identify a 2-furoyl group as the most active antagonist of all tested 2-acylamino-4,6-diphenylpyridine derivatives. They identified compound 9l with an $IC_{50}$ value of 3.7 nM for receptor binding to GPR54 and with high antagonistic activity against KP-10-stimulated intracellular calcium release. Further optimization yielded compound 15a containing a piperazine ring which exhibited high affinity binding to both human and rat GPR54 with $IC_{50}$ values of 3.6 and 15 nM, respectively. Compound 15a exhibited high antagonistic activity against KP-10-stimulated calcium release in CHO cells stably expressing GPR54ß. These antagonists have yet to be studied in man.

*Use of Antagonists to Interrogate the Role of Kisspeptin in Physiology*

The efficacy of antagonists 210 and 234 was established by the demonstration of their ability to inhibit KP stimulation of LH in male rats and mice [23]. Although basal LH was inhibited by GnRH antagonists, KP antagonists did not inhibit basal LH, suggesting a component of GnRH secretion is independent of KP. KP antagonist 234 directly inhibited KP stimulation of GnRH neuron firing in mouse brain slices at low concentration (1 nM) and, in pubertal female rhesus monkeys, 234 inhibited GnRH pulses but not basal levels [23]. This provides direct evidence for a role for KP in GnRH secretion at puberty. In another study in prepubertal female monkeys, GnRH was suppressed for 90 min by 234 suggesting that there is a lower KP tone. Antagonist 234 was also effective in suppressing LH (GnRH) pulsatility in ovariectomized ewes without affecting basal LH [23] and decreased LH pulse frequency, but not basal LH, when administered into the ARC in ovariectomized female rats. Antagonist 234 delayed puberty in female rats, which together with the effects on GnRH pulse frequency in pubertal and prepubertal monkeys confirms a role for KP in puberty; this was also suggested by the failure to progress through puberty in patients with GPR54 and KP mutations [3, 5, 6].

Studies with 234 also demonstrated that KP is required for the elevation of LH when removing negative sex steroid feedback by orchidectomy of sheep and laboratory rodents [23]. The positive feedback of estrogen in the LH ovulatory surge in female rats was also shown directly to be KP dependent as 234 inhibited this surge [23], as was demonstrated with KP antiserum.

Small-molecule KP antagonists such as 15a (fig. 5b) can penetrate the blood-brain barrier. Our group considered the possibility of conveying brain penetration to KP peptides by attaching the penetratin sequence to the amino terminus of 234. This molecule was able to inhibit the LH stimulation by intracerebroventricular KP when it was administered systemically to rats and to inhibit the LH surge in ewes. Thus, KP antagonists are powerful tools for demonstrating the physiological role of KP in GnRH neuron firing and GnRH pulsatility, in positive and negative feedback by gonadal steroids, in the LH surge of ovulation and in puberty. KP antagonists have also highlighted that GnRH secretion is not entirely dependent on KP as basal GnRH and LH were unaffected by KP antagonist in these studies.

In summary, our studies have demonstrated that KP antagonists may be effectively utilized to interrogate the role of KP in the above and other physiological paradigms, such as the effects of leptin, inhibin, activin, follistatin and nutrients, and the dialogue of KP, NKB and dynorphin A in GnRH/LH secretion.

### *Potential Clinical Applications of Kisspeptin Antagonists*

Stimulation of gonadotropin by native KP-54 and KP-10 has been extensively studied in humans. KP-54 stimulated the secretion of gonadotropins in healthy women and in women with hypothalamic amenorrhea. However, long-term treatment induced tachyphylaxis [28]. Administration of KP-54 to premenopausal women with regular menstrual cycles resulted in greater gonadotropin response during the preovulatory phase of the menstrual cycle and minimal response during the follicular phase [29]. Postmenopausal women had a greater LH response to KP-10 than women in the follicular phase of the menstrual cycle and women with progestogen implants, whereas women on the combined contraceptive pill did not have a significant response, indicating a greater degree of negative feedback [30].

Bolus administration of KP-54 or KP-10 to healthy men elicited robust stimulation of gonadotropin secretion [19, 31] and continuous infusion of KP-10 for 22.5 h increased gonadotropin secretion and pulse frequency, with no tachyphylaxis over this period [19]. Continuous KP-10 infusion stimulated robust LH responses in men with type 2 diabetes mellitus, in whom low serum testosterone levels are commonly observed, and restored testosterone levels to within the normal range [32]. These findings suggest that long-acting formulations of KP-10 or synthetic agonists might find utility in men with hypogonadism and for the induction of ovulation in women. On the other hand, the finding that long-term treatment with KP agonists can induce more rapid and profound inhibition of testosterone than the GnRH agonist leuprorelin in male rats suggests that agonists might also be used for steroid hormone ablation to castration levels in the treatment of prostate and possibly breast cancers [26].

Since KP is a major regulator of GnRH but a degree of GnRH secretion is KP independent, KP antagonists might be employed as partial inhibitors of gonadotropin and sex steroids. GnRH analogs have found extensive therapeutic applications in hormone-dependent diseases and in IVF. GnRH agonists induce gonadotrope desensitization while antagonists prevent receptor activation by endogenous GnRH. Both treatments result in suppression of gonadotropin secretion with consequent reduction in circulating gonadal steroid hormones. In these treatments, steroid hormones are lowered to castrate levels resulting in side effects such as hot flushes, reduced lean body mass, loss of libido and bone loss. Our demonstration that KP antagonists reduce LH pulsatility and inhibit the ovulatory LH surge, but do not appear to affect basal LH, suggests that they may find clinical utility in conditions where maximal suppression of sex steroids is contraindicated. Partial sex steroid suppression with KP antagonists may find utility in benign prostatic hyperplasia, endometriosis and uterine fibroids, where lowering of gonadal steroids could improve the conditions without the side effects of reducing steroid hormones to castrate levels. PCOS, which is characterized by increased LH pulse frequency and an increased LH/FSH ratio, is another potential target of KP therapy. Although unproven, lowering of GnRH pulse frequency by KP antagonists should maintain FSH (favored by low pulse frequency) while lowering LH as desired in PCOS. As this would allow follicle development and estrogen production but inhibit ovulation, it may be an attractive possibility as a female contraceptive. KP antagonists may also find application in IVF to prevent premature luteinization while maintaining basal LH, which may be of value in some women during superovulation.

The discovery of KP antagonists provides a new avenue for investigating the role of KP in the normal physiology and pathophysiology of gonadotropin regulation in humans. They also have potentially new therapeutic approaches for the treatment of hormone-dependent diseases without generating the side effects of current therapeutics which induce total ablation of gonadal steroids.

## Neurokinin B Analogs

### *Background*

NKB recently emerged as a novel neuropeptide with a crucial role in the neuroendocrine regulation of reproduction through the identification of inactivating mutations in the genes encoding NKB and its cognate receptor, TACR3/NK3R, which, like KP and GPR54 mutations, result in a failure to progress through puberty and in adult hypogonadotropic hypogonadism [4, 7]. Although inactivation of the NKB system in rodents does not fully replicate human findings, studies in monkeys, goats and sheep show a clear stimulatory role for NKB in gonadotropin secretion, in keeping with the observations in humans of decreased LH in the absence of NKB signaling. The patients with inactivating mutations of genes encoding NKB or its receptor were characterized by very low LH but normal or near-normal circulating FSH levels [4]. This situation would be produced by a low GnRH pulse frequency. In contrast, inactivating mutations in GPR54 result in low levels of both LH and FSH [5, 6]. Thus, it was suggested that a loss of KP signaling leads to a major loss of GnRH pulsatility whilst a loss of NKB signaling leads to low-frequency GnRH pulsatility.

KP neurons in the ARC were shown to co-express NKB and dynorphin A [33] and were therefore named KNDy neurons. Since GnRH neurons express GPR54 but apparently not NK3R, while KNDy neurons express NK3R, it was further postulated that NKB secreted from KNDy neurons acts in an autocrine or paracrine manner to enhance KP secretion and that NKB actions were upstream of KP [34]. The demonstration that continuous infusion of KP at a GPR54-saturating concentration in patients with NKB- or NK3R-inactivating mutations restored LH pulsatility provided strong support for this notion [34].

The positioning of NKB actions upstream of KP and GnRH raises the possibility that modulation of NKB signaling with agonists and antagonists will be more subtle than modulation of KP signaling, which in turn is more subtle than modulation of GnRH signaling. This being the case, there are distinct opportunities for the development and utilization of drugs which target the three levels of the neuroendocrine cascade with differential effects on gonadotropin and steroid hormones. Analogs of NKB and their potential therapeutic applications are considered below.

### *Neurokinin B Analogs*

NKB is a decapeptide (fig. 6) cleaved from a prepro precursor protein. It is a member of the tachykinin family of peptides which are characterized by a common carboxyl-terminal motif: Phe-X-Gly-Leu-Met-$NH_2$. NKB interacts with all three mammalian tachykinin receptors (TACR1, TACR2 and TACR3/NK3R) but has highest selectivity for NK3R, which couples principally through $G_{q/11}$ G proteins.

The majority of the hundreds of patented molecules show selectivity for TACR1 or TACR2, but a few analogs have been developed which are highly selective for TACR3/NK3R. Because the role of NKB in the neuroendocrine control of reproduction is a relatively recent discovery, the therapeutic targets for NK3R-selective antagonists have generally been in the CNS field (e.g. schizophrenia, anxiety, pain and inflammation) and also in some pulmonary (e.g. chronic obstructive pulmonary disease) and gastrointestinal tract (e.g. irritable bowel syndrome) diseases. Since NK3R antagonists were largely ineffective in these conditions, there is a huge opportunity to exploit these analogs in delineating the role of NKB in reproduction and as potential therapeutics in the area.

The first NK3R-selective peptide agonist analog, senktide (selective neurokinin B receptor peptide), was developed by systematic methylation of the peptide bonds in a truncated version of the TACR1-selective tachykinin, substance P (fig. 6) [35]. This modified peptide also had much higher metabolic stability than the native tachykinins, making it a useful experimental tool. An analog of the NKB in which the $Val^7$ has been replaced with MePhe [$MePhe^7$]NKB, (fig. 6) or Pro retains high affinity for NK3R and improved selectivity for tachykinin receptors.

Several, non-peptide NK3R-selective antagonists have also been developed. These fall into two main structural classes: dichlorophenylalkylpiperidines (e.g. osanetant)

| | | |
|---|---|---|
| | NKB: | Asp — Met — His — Asp — Phe — Phe — Val — Gly — Leu — Met — $NH_2$ |
| | Senktide: | Succinyl — Asp — Phe — MePhe — Gly — Leu — Met — $NH_2$ |
| **a** | [MePhe$^7$]NKB: | Asp — Met — His — Asp — Phe — Phe — MePhe — Gly — Leu — Met — $NH_2$ |

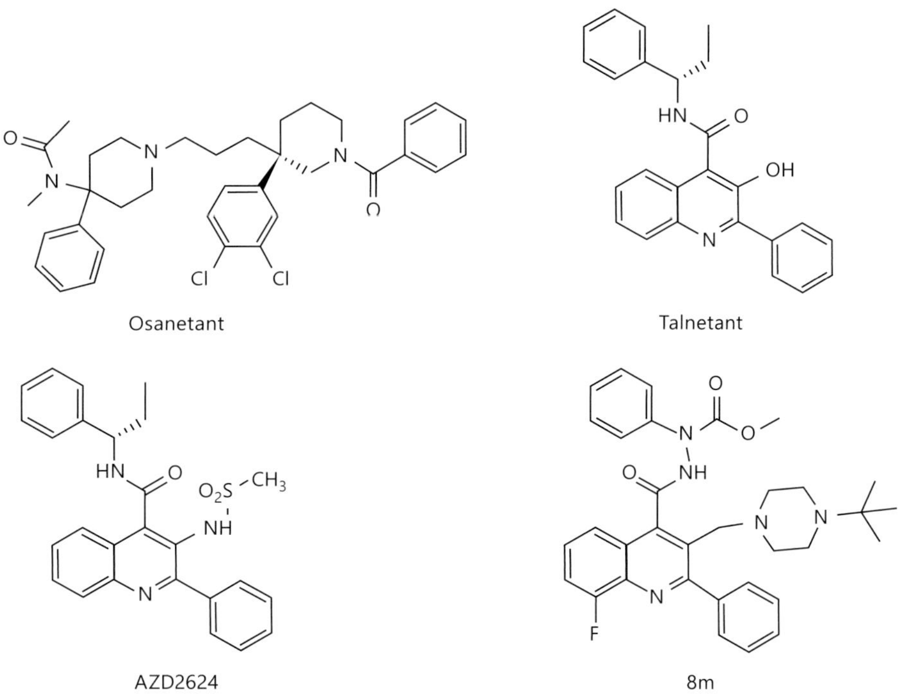


**b**

**Fig. 6.** NKB analogs. **a** Peptide agonist analogs specific for NK3R. Senktide is an analog of substance P which is highly selective for NK3R whilst [MePhe$^7$]NKB is not as selective for NK3R and can also activate TACR2 at high concentrations. **b** Nonpeptide antagonists highly selective for NK3R. Osanetant, talnetant and AZD2624 have all been tested in humans for nonreproductive applications. Thus, proof-of-concept reproductive studies would be insightful. The compound 8m has not yet entered the clinic. Reproduced from Millar and Newton [8].

and quinolones (e.g. talnetant). Osanetant (SR142801; fig. 6) was developed by modification of the TACR2 receptor-selective compound saredutant, and was the first high-affinity nonpeptide NK3R-selective antagonist to be described. Modified analogs of osanetant, including SSR-146997, have since been developed. Differentially substituted 4-quinoline carboxamides have also been identified as TACR3-selective antagonists which displayed similar potency but increased NK3R selectivity compared to osanetant. Modifications to optimize these initial compounds led to the identification of talnetant (SB-223412), an orally active, potent and selective NK3R antagonist. Analogs of talnetant with increased blood-brain barrier permeability (SB-222200 and GSK256471) or no blood-brain barrier permeability (SB-335375) have since been described. SB-222200 is problematic as a research tool in view of its very poor solubility. Other talnetant-based TACR3 antagonists have also been developed including AZD2624 and the N′2-diphenylquinoline-4-carbohydrazide Merck compound 8m.

Although TACR3 antagonists had not been clinically tested for reproductive effects, osanetant, talnetant and AZD2624 have been subject to clinical trials assessing their effectiveness in treating CNS disorders (e.g. schizophrenia, anxiety and depression) and other non-CNS indications (e.g. irritable bowel syndrome or overactive bladder). The efficacy was inconclusive and clinical development of most of these NK3R antagonists for the treatment of CNS disorders has been discontinued.

### *Potential Therapeutic Applications of Neurokinin B Analogs*

The development of NKB agonists and antagonists has potential in therapeutic interventions in various dysfunctions of the reproductive system. As mentioned earlier, the upstream position of NKB suggests that analogs will have less complete effects than KP analogs, which in turn will have less complete effects than GnRH analogs. Consequently, NKB antagonists or densensitization with agonists will potentially be less effective in lowering LH and have little effect on FSH as is evident in patients with deficiencies in NKB signaling. These analogs are therefore unlikely to be of value in treating hormone-dependent cancers, such as prostatic cancer, in which lowering of sex steroids to castration levels is a prerequisite for efficacy, as accomplished with GnRH analogs. However, this property of reduced lowering of LH is likely to be valuable in conditions which require partial inhibition of sex steroids and the avoidance of side effects such as bone loss, loss of libido and hot flushes, which are characteristic of GnRH analog treatment.

NKB antagonists mimic inactivating mutations of human NKB and NK3R in reducing LH pulse frequency and amplitude without affecting FSH, and are therefore likely to be efficacious in treating PCOS, which is characterized by elevated LH pulse frequency and amplitude along with an increased LH/FSH ratio [36]. NKB antagonists appear also to have potential in novel female contraception as disruption of NKB signaling maintains FSH (and estradiol) but decreases LH, and therefore would potentially prevent ovulation. NKB antagonists are likely to lower LH to a lesser degree than KP antagonists and may be even more suitable for partial suppression of gonadotropins and gonadal steroids in hormone-dependent diseases, such as endometriosis and benign prostatic hyperplasia, without inducing bone loss or hot flushes.

In conditions of decreased LH production and near normal FSH secretion (i.e. due to low GnRH pulse frequency) such as hypothalamic amenorrhea or delayed puberty [28], restoration of LH and normal reproductive function may potentially be achieved by treatment with NKB (or KP) agonists. NKB agonists may also find utility in a more gentle stimulation of gonadotropins in assisted reproduction technologies as suggested for KP. However, a potential limitation in the therapeutic use of NKB agonists is tachyphylaxis, which has been reported in monkeys [37]. Tachyphylaxis was also observed in long-term administration of KP-54 to women with hypothalamic amenorrhea [28] and in monkeys [38]. However, this may be an issue of time and dose as tachyphylaxis was not observed in men receiving continuous infusion of KP-10 at near-maximal LH-stimulating levels over 22 h [19].

## Potential Applications of Novel Hypothalamic Neuropeptide Analogs in Precocious Puberty

The treatment of precocious puberty with GnRH agonist analogs was a superb breakthrough in ameliorating this vexing condition such that the advance in puberty could be halted indefinitely until such time as it was appropriate to withdraw treatment and allow progress through puberty. However, the treatment results in a total suppression of sex steroids and it is reasonable to pose the question 'should patients not be exposed to low levels of sex steroids for normal development?' This may be achieved in several ways:

- Replacement of low-level sex steroids while receiving GnRH agonist
- Provision of low-level sex steroids in the form of GnRH analog-steroid conjugates
- Use of KP or NKB analogs to partially suppress gonadotropins

Animal studies to examine the benefits of these alternatives will be instructive.

## Conclusions

Reproductive hormones play important roles at all stages of development from gamete production and fertilization, through puberty and adulthood to senescence. The hormone cascades of brain neuroendocrine peptides, gonadotropins and steroid hormones are all targets for the development of analogs for intervention in normal physiological and pathophysiological processes. Orally active GnRH analogs, bifunctional GnRH analog-steroid conjugates and the arrival of novel neuroendocrine analogs of KP and NKB increase therapeutic options, and their more proximal position in the cascade holds promise for more subtle interventions in pediatric and adult medicine.

## Acknowledgments

We acknowledge support from the Medical Research Council (South Africa), the National Research Foundation, the University of Pretoria, the Claude Leon Trust and the University of Cape Town.

## References


1 Millar RP, Lu ZL, Pawson AJ, Flanagan CA, Morgan K, Maudsley SR: Gonadotropin-releasing hormone receptors. Endocr Rev 2004;25:235–275.

2 Millar RP: GnRHs and GnRH receptors. Anim Reprod Sci 2005;88:5–28.

3 Topaloglu AK, Tello JA, Kotan LD, Ozbek MN, Yilmaz MB, Erdogan S, Gurbuz F, Temiz F, Millar RP, Yuksel B: Inactivating KISS1 mutation and hypogonadotropic hypogonadism. N Engl J Med 2012;366:629–635.

4 Topaloglu AK, Reimann F, Guclu M, Yalin AS, Kotan LD, Porter KM, Serin A, Mungan NO, Cook JR, Ozbek MN, Imamoglu S, Akalin NS, Yuksel B, O'Rahilly S, Semple RK: TAC3 and TACR3 mutations in familial hypogonadotropic hypogonadism reveal a key role for neurokinin B in the central control of reproduction. Nat Genet 2009;41:354–358.

5 Seminara SB, Messager S, Chatzidaki EE, Thresher RR, Acierno JS Jr, Shagoury JK, Bo-Abbas Y, Kuohung W, Schwinof KM, Hendrick AG, Zahn D, Dixon J, Kaiser UB, Slaugenhaupt SA, Gusella JF, O'Rahilly S, Carlton MB, Crowley WF Jr, Aparicio SA, Colledge WH: The GPR54 gene as a regulator of puberty. N Engl J Med 2003;349:1614–1627.

6 de Roux N, Genin E, Carel JC, Matsuda F, Chaussain JL, Milgrom E: Hypogonadotropic hypogonadism due to loss of function of the KiSS1-derived peptide receptor GPR54. Proc Natl Acad Sci U S A 2003;100:10972–10976.

7 Young J, Bouligand J, Francou B, Raffin-Sanson ML, Gaillez S, Jeanpierre M, Grynberg M, Kamenicky P, Chanson P, Brailly-Tabard S, Guiochon-Mantel A: TAC3 and TACR3 defects cause hypothalamic congenital hypogonadotropic hypogonadism in humans. J Clin Endocrinol Metab 2010;95:2287–2295.

8 Millar RP, Newton CL: Current and future applications of GnRH, kisspeptin and neurokinin B analogues. Nat Rev Endocrinol 2013;9:451–466.

9 King JA, Millar RP: Heterogeneity of vertebrate luteinizing hormone-releasing hormone. Science 1979;206:67–69.

10 King JA, Millar RP: Structure of chicken hypothalamic luteinizing hormone-releasing hormone. I. Structural determination on partially purified material. J Biol Chem 1982;257:10722.

11 Sherwood NM, Lovejoy DA, Coe IR: Origin of mammalian gonadotropin-releasing hormones. Endocr Rev 1993;14:241–254.

12 Karten MJ, Rivier JE: Gonadotropin-releasing hormone analog design. Structure-function studies toward the development of agonists and antagonists: rationale and perspective. Endocr Rev 1986;7:44–66.

13 Ratcliffe KE, Fraser HM, Sellar R, Rivier J, Millar RP: Bifunctional gonadotropin-releasing hormone antagonist-progesterone analogs with increased efficacy and duration of action. Endocrinology 2006;147:571–579.

14 Conn PM, Ulloa-Aguirre A: Pharmacological chaperones for misfolded gonadotropin-releasing hormone receptors. Adv Pharmacol 2011;62:109–141.

15 Tsutsumi M, Zhou W, Millar RP, Mellon PL, Roberts JL, Flanagan CA, Dong K, Gillo B, Sealfon SC: Cloning and functional expression of a mouse gonadotropin-releasing hormone receptor. Mol Endocrinol 1992;6:1163–1169.

16 Millar RP, Pawson AJ, Morgan K, Rissman EF, Lu ZL: Diversity of actions of GnRHs mediated by ligand-induced selective signaling. Front Neuroendocrinol 2008;29:17–35.

17 Lahlou N, Roger M, Chaussain JL, Feinstein MC, Sultan C, Toublanc JE, Schally AV, Scholler R: Gonadotropin and alpha-subunit secretion during long term pituitary suppression by D-Trp6-luteinizing hormone-releasing hormone microcapsules as treatment of precocious puberty. J Clin Endocrinol Metab 1987;65:946–953.

18 Roseweir AK, Millar RP: The role of kisspeptin in the control of gonadotrophin secretion. Hum Reprod Update 2009;15:203–212.

19 George JT, Veldhuis JD, Roseweir AK, Newton CL, Faccenda E, Millar RP, Anderson RA: Kisspeptin-10 is a potent stimulator of LH and increases pulse frequency in men. J Clin Endocrinol Metab 2011;96:E1228–E1236.

20 Ratnasabapathy R, Dhillo WS: The effects of kisspeptin in human reproductive function – therapeutic implications. Curr Drug Targets 2013;14:365–371.

21 Oakley AE, Clifton DK, Steiner RA: Kisspeptin signaling in the brain. Endocr Rev 2009;30:713–743.

22 Pinilla L, Aguilar E, Dieguez C, Millar RP, Tena-Sempere M: Kisspeptins and reproduction: physiological roles and regulatory mechanisms. Physiol Rev 2012;92:1235–1316.

23 Roseweir AK, Kauffman AS, Smith JT, Guerriero KA, Morgan K, Pielecka-Fortuna J, Pineda R, Gottsch ML, Tena-Sempere M, Moenter SM, Terasawa E, Clarke IJ, Steiner RA, Millar RP: Discovery of potent kisspeptin antagonists delineate physiological mechanisms of gonadotropin regulation. J Neurosci 2009;29:3920–3929.

24 Asami T, Nishizawa N: Metastin derivatives and use thereof. Patent No. US 7960348 B2. Osaka, Takeda Pharmaceutical Company Limited, 2011.

25 Kitada C, Asami T, Nishizawa N: Metastin derivatives and use thereof. Patent No. US 7625869. Osaka, Takeda Pharmaceutical Company Limited, 2009.

26 Matsui H, Tanaka A, Yokoyama K, Takatsu Y, Ishikawa K, Asami T, Nishizawa N, Suzuki A, Kumano S, Terada M, Kusaka M, Kitada C, Ohtaki T: Chronic administration of the metastin/kisspeptin analog KISS1-305 or the investigational agent TAK-448 suppresses hypothalamic pituitary gonadal function and depletes plasma testosterone in adult male rats. Endocrinology 2012;153:5297–5308.
27 Kobayashi T, Sasaki S, Tomita N, Fukui S, Kuroda N, Nakayama M, Kiba A, Takatsu Y, Ohtaki T, Itoh F, Baba A: Synthesis and structure-activity relationships of 2-acylamino-4,6-diphenylpyridine derivatives as novel antagonists of GPR54. Bioorg Med Chem 2010;18:3841–3859.
28 Jayasena CN, Nijher GM, Chaudhri OB, Murphy KG, Ranger A, Lim A, Patel D, Mehta A, Todd C, Ramachandran R, Salem V, Stamp GW, Donaldson M, Ghatei MA, Bloom SR, Dhillo WS: Subcutaneous injection of kisspeptin-54 acutely stimulates gonadotropin secretion in women with hypothalamic amenorrhea, but chronic administration causes tachyphylaxis. J Clin Endocrinol Metab 2009;94: 4315–4323.
29 Dhillo WS, Chaudhri OB, Thompson EL, Murphy KG, Patterson M, Ramachandran R, Nijher GK, Amber V, Kokkinos A, Donaldson M, Ghatei MA, Bloom SR: Kisspeptin-54 stimulates gonadotropin release most potently during the preovulatory phase of the menstrual cycle in women. J Clin Endocrinol Metab 2007;92:3958–3966.
30 George JT, Anderson RA, Millar RP: Kisspeptin-10 stimulation of gonadotrophin secretion in women is modulated by sex steroid feedback. Hum Reprod 2012;27:3552–3559.
31 Dhillo WS, Chaudhri OB, Patterson M, Thompson EL, Murphy KG, Badman MK, McGowan BM, Amber V, Patel S, Ghatei MA, Bloom SR: Kisspeptin-54 stimulates the hypothalamic-pituitary gonadal axis in human males. J Clin Endocrinol Metab 2005;90: 6609–6615.
32 George JT, Veldhuis JD, Tena-Sempere M, Millar RP, Anderson RA: Exploring the pathophysiology of hypogonadism in men with type 2 diabetes: kisspeptin-10 stimulates serum testosterone and LH secretion in men with type 2 diabetes and mild biochemical hypogonadism. Clin Endocrinol 2013;79: 100–104.
33 Goodman RL, Lehman MN, Smith JT, Coolen LM, de Oliveira CV, Jafarzadehshirazi MR, Pereira A, Iqbal J, Caraty A, Ciofi P, Clarke IJ: Kisspeptin neurons in the arcuate nucleus of the ewe express both dynorphin A and neurokinin B. Endocrinology 2007;148:5752–5760.
34 Young J, George JT, Tello JA, Francou B, Bouligand J, Guiochon-Mantel A, Brailly-Tabard S, Anderson RA, Millar RP: Kisspeptin restores pulsatile LH secretion in patients with neurokinin B signaling deficiencies: physiological, pathophysiological and therapeutic implications. Neuroendocrinology 2013;97: 193–202.
35 Wormser U, Laufer R, Hart Y, Chorev M, Gilon C, Selinger Z: Highly selective agonists for substance P receptor subtypes. EMBO J 1986;5:2805–2808.
36 Blank SK, McCartney CR, Marshall JC: The origins and sequelae of abnormal neuroendocrine function in polycystic ovary syndrome. Hum Reprod Update 2006;12:351–361.
37 Ramaswamy S, Seminara SB, Plant TM: Evidence from the agonadal juvenile male rhesus monkey *(Macaca mulatta)* for the view that the action of neurokinin B to trigger gonadotropin-releasing hormone release is upstream from the kisspeptin receptor. Neuroendocrinology 2011;94:237–245.
38 Seminara SB, Dipietro MJ, Ramaswamy S, Crowley WF Jr, Plant TM: Continuous human metastin 45–54 infusion desensitizes G protein-coupled receptor 54-induced gonadotropin-releasing hormone release monitored indirectly in the juvenile male rhesus monkey *(Macaca mulatta)*: a finding with therapeutic implications. Endocrinology 2006;147:2122–2126.

Robert P. Millar, PhD, FRSE
The Mammal Research Institute
Department of Zoology and Entomology
Faculty of Natural and Agricultural Sciences
University of Pretoria
Lynwood Road, Hatfield, Pretoria 0028 (South Africa)
E-Mail robertpetermillar@gmail.com

Cappa M, Cianfarani S, Ghizzoni L, Loche S, Maghnie M (eds): Advanced Therapies in Pediatric Endocrinology and Diabetology. Endocr Dev. Basel, Karger, 2016, vol 30, pp 130–140 (DOI: 10.1159/000439338)

# Aromatase Inhibitors in the Treatment of Short Stature

Matti Hero

Children's Hospital, Helsinki University Central Hospital (HUCH), Helsinki, Finland

**Abstract**

Reports published in the 1990s of men with estrogen deficiency caused by defective aromatase or estrogen resistance due to a defective estrogen receptor α confirmed the crucial role of estrogen in bone maturation, closure of the epiphyses and cessation of statural growth. Based on these findings, it became reasonable to postulate that selective inhibition of estrogen synthesis with aromatase inhibitors could increase adult height by delaying bone maturation and prolonging the period of growth in males. To date, aromatase inhibitors have been employed in rare pediatric conditions associated with sex steroid excess, and in randomized controlled trials involving boys with short stature and/or constitutional delay of puberty. Findings from these randomized trials suggest that potent aromatase inhibitors increase predicted height, but final adult height data are scarce. Moreover, several safety issues remain inadequately studied. In this paper, published findings on the use of aromatase inhibitors in growth indications are reviewed with emphasis on treatment efficacy and safety.



Aromatase is the key enzyme that converts androgens to estrogens, specifically androstenedione to estrone and testosterone to estradiol. Aromatase and estrogen receptors are expressed in several tissues and cell types in males and females, suggesting a diverse role for estrogen also at sites outside the hypothalamus-pituitary-gonadal axis [1]. The expression of aromatase is regulated in a tissue-specific manner by specific promoters in different tissues [1].

Reports published in the 1990s of men with either estrogen deficiency caused by defective aromatase or estrogen resistance due to defective estrogen receptor α confirmed the crucial role of estrogen in bone maturation, closure of the epiphyses and cessation of statural growth [2–4]. Based on these findings, it became reasonable to postulate that selective inhibition of estrogen synthesis or action could increase adult height by delaying bone maturation and prolonging the period of growth in males. To date, aromatase inhibitors – blockers of estrogen biosynthesis – have been used in several different pediatric conditions associated with sex steroid excess or poor adult height prognosis [for review, please see ref. 5]. Previous reports have shown that aromatase inhibitor treatment normalizes growth velocity and the rate of bone maturation, and increases predicted adult height in boys with testotoxicosis [6, 7]. Based on case reports, aromatase inhibitors are also probably effective in males with rare conditions associated with estrogen excess [8–10]. In contrast, these compounds have shown only partial efficacy in girls with McCune-Albright syndrome [11, 12], and inefficacy in males with pubertal gynecomastia [13]. Aromatase inhibitors have also been used in combination with an antiandrogen in children with congenital adrenal hyperplasia, but at present published data from controlled studies in this patient group are very limited [14].

After a short introduction to aromatase inhibitors, published findings on the use of aromatase inhibitors in the treatment of short stature and/or constitutional delay of growth and puberty (CDGP) are reviewed, with emphasis on treatment efficacy and safety.

## Aromatase Inhibitors

Aromatase inhibitors are a class of compounds that inhibit the aromatase either competitively (nonsteroidal compounds) or by covalently binding to the active site of the aromatase enzyme (steroidal compounds) [15]. The first aromatase inhibitor on the market was aminoglutethimide, which required four times daily dosing and had significant toxicity. Subsequently, the first generation aromatase inhibitors (aminoglutethimide and testolactone) were replaced by second generation compounds and, more recently, third generation compounds that are almost completely selective and highly potent, and allow once daily dosing due to their longer half-life. Based on studies in postmenopausal women, modern third generation compounds inhibit estrogen biosynthesis by more than 97% (table 1). Most of the recent pediatric studies have been performed with the nonsteroidal third generation aromatase inhibitors anastrozole and letrozole.

A pharmacodynamic study with anastrozole (0.5 or 1 mg/day) in adolescent boys showed that, at least in the short term, the treatment is not associated with significant changes in protein synthesis and kinetically measured rates or indirect markers of bone calcium turnover [16]. No pharmacological studies have been performed with letrozole in adolescents. However, based on the level of stimulation of gonadotropin secretion, letrozole 2.5 mg/day appears to be more potent than anastrozole 1 mg/day [17].

**Table 1.** Classification of aromatase inhibitors

| Generation | Nonsteroidal | Steroidal | Suppression of estrogen production, %[a] |
|---|---|---|---|
| 1st | Aminoglutethimide (250 mg 4 times daily) | | 90.6 |
| | | Testolactone (125 mg twice daily) | <90.6 |
| 2nd | Fadrozole (2 mg twice daily) | | 92.6 |
| | | Formestane (125 mg twice daily) | 91.9 |
| 3rd | Anastrozole (1 mg/day) | | 97.3 |
| | Letrozole (2.5 mg/day) | | >99.1 |
| | Vorozole (2.5 mg/day) | | 89 |
| | | Exemestane (25 mg/day) | 98 |

[a] Data from Geffner et al. [39].

## Aromatase Inhibitors in the Treatment of Short Stature and Constitutional Delay of Growth and Puberty

The aromatase inhibitor letrozole has been used in three randomized placebo-controlled trials involving boys with idiopathic short stature (ISS) [18] or CDGP [19, 20], and anastrozole has been given in combination with growth hormone (GH) in a randomized placebo-controlled study of GH-deficient boys [21]. In addition, first year results of a study involving short boys randomized to receive either anastrozole or letrozole were published recently [17]. Altogether, these randomized clinical studies have included 122 boys treated with aromatase inhibitors for a duration of 1–3 years. As regards predicted adult height, all the studies have reported favorable responses to aromatase inhibitor treatment in the short term, whereas differences exist in the maintenance of the treatment response (table 2). Significant differences in baseline characteristics of the patients were evident between the ISS [18] and the CDGP [19, 20] studies (table 2).

### *Treatment Impact on Estradiol Synthesis and the Hypothalamus-Pituitary-Gonadal Axis*

In the Finnish randomized trials employing letrozole, serum estradiol levels were measured using ultrasensitive radioimmunoassays, with a detection level of 4.5 pmol/l [18, 19]. In both studies, in letrozole-treated boys, circulating estradiol levels remained

**Table 2.** Outcome in published randomized placebo-controlled trials of aromatase inhibitor treatment in boys with ISS or CDGP

| | Wickman et al. [19][a] | | | Hero et al. [18] | | | Salehpour et al. [20] | | |
|---|---|---|---|---|---|---|---|---|---|
| | letrozole | placebo | p | letrozole | placebo | p | letrozole | placebo | p |
| *Treatment duration, months* | 12 | 12 | | 24 | 24 | | 24 | 24 | |
| *Baseline characteristics* | | | | | | | | | |
| Subjects, n | 11 | 12 | | 16 | 14 | | 31 | 30 | |
| Age, years | 15.2 | 15.0 | n.s. | 11.0 | 11.0 | n.s. | 13.6 | 13.5 | |
| Height, SDS | –1.8 | –2.0 | n.s. | –2.3 | –2.4 | n.s. | –2.9 | –2.9 | |
| Genital stage of puberty | 2 (2–3) | 2 (2–3) | n.s. | 1 (1–3) | 1 (1–2) | n.s. | 1 | 1 | |
| Bone age, years | 13.1 | 12.6 | n.s. | 9.1 | 8.9 | n.s. | 12.1 | 11.7 | |
| *Outcome* | | | | | | | | | |
| ΔBone age/Δcalendar age during treatment | 0.6[b] | 1.1[b] | <0.05 | 0.6 | 1.0 | <0.05 | 0.55 | 0.25 | <0.001 |
| PAH, cm | | | | | | | | | |
| Change during the treatment | 5.1[b] | 0.3[b] | <0.05 | 5.9 | 1.1 | <0.01 | 6.1 | 1.4 | NA |
| After treatment[c] | NA | NA | | 166.5 | 162.4 | 0.57 | NA | NA | |
| Near-final height, cm[d] | 175.8 | 169.1 | <0.05 | NA | NA | | NA | NA | |
| Final adult height, cm[e] | 177.6 | 170.1 | 0.06 | NA | NA | | NA | NA | |

PAH = Predicted adult height; NA = not available.
[a] Letrozole or placebo in combination with low-dose testosterone for 6 months.
[b] Evaluated 6 months after treatment cessation.
[c] Evaluated 4.2 years after treatment cessation.
[d] Near-final height was determined by bone age ≥15.75 years: n = 9 (letrozole group) and n = 8 (placebo group).
[e] At final adult height: n = 6 (letrozole group) and n = 6 (placebo group).

at the low pretreatment level despite significant increases in testosterone level and progression of signs of puberty, indicating significant inhibition of estrogen biosynthesis. In the study of boys with ISS, serum estradiol remained low in boys who progressed in puberty despite a mean serum testosterone concentration of 30.9 nmol/l 24 months after treatment onset [18]. In the study by Wickman et al. [19] including boys with more advanced stage of puberty, mean serum estradiol remained equally low, despite an even higher mean testosterone level of 50.9 nmol/l after 12 months of treatment with an equal dose of letrozole (2.5 mg/day). At the same time, in both placebo-controlled studies, serum gonadotropin levels were significantly higher in those randomized to receive letrozole. Thus, letrozole effectively inhibits estrogen biosynthesis in adolescent boys, decreases the estrogen-mediated negative feedback effect on gonadotropin secretion and thereby increases testosterone level. In more detail, blockade of estrogen biosynthesis with letrozole appears to increase the pulse amplitude of luteinizing hormone with no clear effect on the frequency of pulses [22]. Interestingly, in adolescent boys, anastrozole has less effect on gonadotropin secretion and circulating testosterone levels [21]. This finding was replicated in the recent study by Neely et al. [17], and it is explained by the lower potency of the compound as compared with letrozole (table 1). Despite the supraphysiological increase in testosterone concentrations in many adolescent boys treated with letrozole, severe androgenic adverse effects have not been reported [17–19]. Hemoglobin concentration in the blood increases in correlation with serum testosterone, but no thrombotic events have been reported [23].

### *Influence on Predicted Adult Height*

In all four placebo-controlled randomized trials of aromatase inhibitor treatment in boys with short stature and/or CDGP, blockade of estrogen biosynthesis decreased the rate of bone maturation with no untoward effect on growth velocity [18–21]. As a result, predicted adult height increased by 5.1–6.7 cm during 1–3 years of therapy, significantly more than in those who received placebo (table 2). It is of note that pubertal boys treated with aromatase inhibitors showed pubertal growth velocities despite of prepubertal insulin-like growth factor 1 (IGF-1) levels, supporting the view that androgens have direct growth-enhancing effects in adolescent boys [18, 19].

### *Influence on Near-Final Height and Final Adult Height*

In general, posttreatment follow-up data from placebo-controlled studies of aromatase inhibitor treatment in patients with short stature and/or CDGP are scarce. However, the boys with CDGP treated with testosterone (for 6 months) in combination with letrozole or placebo (for 12 months) were evaluated at near-final height recently [24]. Boys treated with testosterone plus placebo reached the mean near-final height of 169.1 cm, while the mean near-final height of boys treated with the testosterone-letrozole combination was 175.8 cm (fig. 1a). The difference in near-final height between the groups was statistically significant. While the near-final height of boys treated with the testosterone-placebo combination was significantly lower than their mid-parental target height, the near-final height of the testosterone-letrozole-treated boys was not (fig. 1a). Twelve patients from this study have been evaluated at final adult height, and it appears that those who received letrozole ended up slightly taller than those who received placebo (table 2). However, in boys with ISS treated with letrozole or placebo for 2 years, the achieved gain in predicted adult height over the placebo group had decreased during later posttreatment growth and maturation; 4.2 years after cessation of treatment no significant difference in predicted adult height between the letrozole group and the placebo group remained (fig. 1b) [25]. This difference in longer-term treatment efficacy between the CDGP and ISS populations can potentially be explained by the younger age and bone age in the latter at cessation of treatment. In fact, a significant proportion of the ISS boys were still prepubertal at the end of the treatment period.

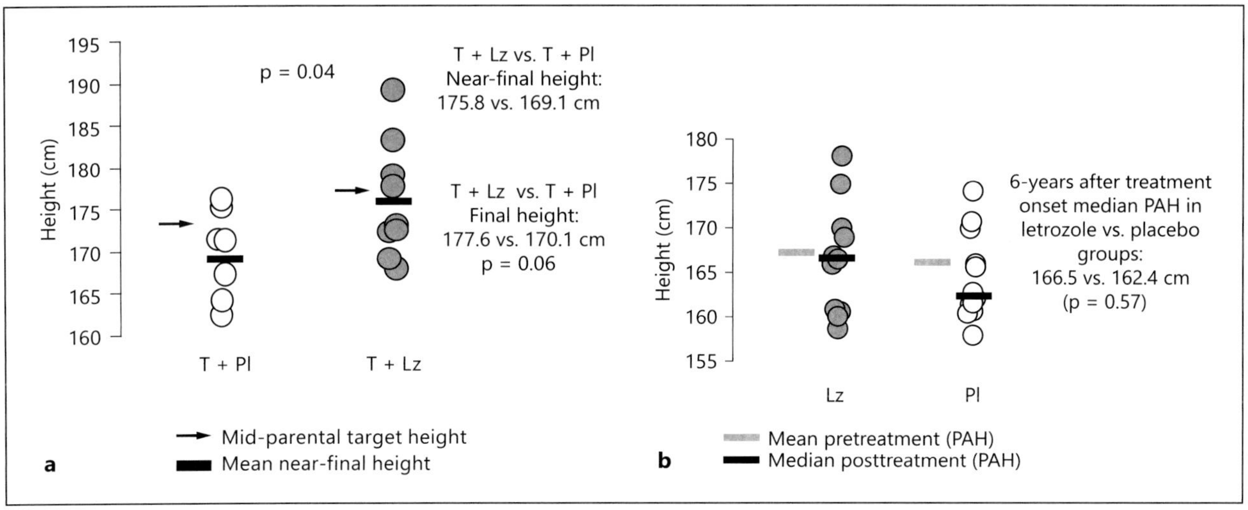


**Fig. 1. a** Near-final height in boys with CDGP treated with testosterone (T) for 6 months in combination with letrozole (Lz) or placebo (Pl) for 12 months. **b** Posttreatment predicted adult height in boys with ISS treated with letrozole (Lz) or placebo (Pl) for 2 years. Approximately half of the boys remained prepubertal during the treatment, and the rest progressed in puberty. PAH = Predicted adult height; T = testosterone.

## Safety of Aromatase Inhibitor Treatment

Supporting an important role for estrogen signaling in human physiology, estrogen receptors and aromatase enzymes are expressed in several different cell types. Therefore, aromatase inhibition may also have unwanted effects in several tissues. Several safety issues, such as the effects of treatment on bone mineral density (BMD), bone turnover, lipid metabolism, insulin sensitivity and cognitive performance, have been addressed in randomized controlled trials employing aromatase inhibitors in boys with short stature and/or CDGP.

### *Bone Health*

Case reports of men with congenital estrogen deficiency support the view that estrogen is important in the accrual and maintenance of bone mass in males [2–4]. Interventional studies employing aromatase inhibitors suggest that estrogen preserves bone mass by inhibiting bone resorption [26]. However, when BMD was followed up with dual-energy X-ray absorptiometry (DXA) in three controlled trials on letrozole treatment in adolescent boys, areal BMD increased in a similar fashion in aromatase inhibitor- and placebo-treated patients [18–20]. Similarly, in a study by Mauras et al. [21], 3-year treatment with anastrozole in combination with GH had no adverse influence on areal BMD in GH-deficient boys compared with placebo and GH. This neutral effect on BMD may be explained by bone-protective effects of elevated androgen levels. In support of this, testosterone appears to stimulate periosteal bone expansion [27]. However, DXA is a 2-dimensional method of assessing bone quantity and gives no data on the effects of aromatase inhibition on bone geometry or quality. Currently, no studies on the effects of sex hormone-modulatory treatments on bone geometry or quantity in different bone compartments of adolescents have been reported.

Recently, vertebral body morphology was evaluated by MRI in a posttreatment study of males previously treated with letrozole either for CDGP or ISS [25]. In men with CDGP treated with letrozole for 1 year during early or mid-puberty, no adverse effects on vertebral morphology were found. However, in males with ISS treated with letrozole for 2 years (in most cases prior to significant pubertal progression), an increased prevalence of mild anterior wedging or compression deformities of the vertebral bodies were found. These findings were not associated with symptoms, and their clinical significance is unclear.

### *Metabolic Parameters*

Aromatase inhibitor treatment of adolescent males has not been associated with adverse influence on LDL cholesterol, triglycerides or apolipoprotein B levels in randomized controlled trials [20, 21, 28, 29]. In contrast, HDL cholesterol decreased by approximately 0.5 mmol/l in pubertal boys receiving letrozole [29]. This transient decline in HDL cholesterol correlated negatively with the treatment-induced increase in serum testosterone. This androgen-mediated decline in HDL cholesterol appears to be related to letrozole treatment only, since anastrozole treatment has not been associated with changes in HDL cholesterol [21].

Treatment with a potent aromatase inhibitor during puberty in males results in a hormonal milieu characterized by normal to high testosterone concentration, low estradiol concentration and low IGF-1 concentration [18, 19]. As evaluated by fasting serum insulin and the homeostasis model assessment index, the effect of these hormonal changes on insulin sensitivity are either neutral [29] or beneficial [28]. Taken together, these findings suggest that preventing the pubertal activation of the GH-IGF-1 axis with aromatase inhibitor also prevents the GH-mediated emergence of pubertal insulin resistance to some degree.

### *Cognitive Function*

Several lines of evidence suggest that estrogen participates in the regulation of cognitive function, particularly in verbal memory processes [30, 31]. This raises the concern that aromatase inhibition during childhood or adolescence might impair cognitive functions. However, when a selection of cognitive tests, focusing on memory function, was included in the follow-up of boys with ISS treated with letrozole or placebo for 2 years, no differences in verbal and spatial performance were found [32]. Similarly, in tests of verbal, working and visuospatial memory, no differences between the groups were evident. In particular, verbal memory function appeared to improve similarly during the study in letrozole and placebo groups. These findings suggest that suppression of estrogen biosynthesis in adolescent males has no significant adverse effect on cognitive performance. However, taking the nature of cognitive testing in children and adolescents at this age and the small sample size into account, it is clear that further studies on this issue are needed.

### *Maturing Spermatogenesis*

Based on animal data, there is concern that aromatase inhibitor treatment may impair fertility in males. Aromatase-knockout male mice show impaired fertility at an older age, and letrozole treatment of male monkeys has resulted in reduced sperm counts and quality [33, 34]. Moreover, many of the male cases of aromatase deficiency have been reported to be infertile. In men, aromatase has also been detected in sperm, and it seems that estrogen produced locally in the sperm may influence the sperm fertilizing capacity [35]. On the other hand, several reports have shown that aromatase inhibitor treatment of subfertile men improves sperm parameters [36, 37]. Arguing against significant adverse effects on spermatogenesis in adolescent males, letrozole treatment of boys with CDGP or ISS did not adversely influence serum inhibin B or testicular growth [18, 19]. To date, only one study has evaluated sperm parameters after aromatase inhibitor treatment during adolescence. In that study, adolescent boys had received anastrozole for 1 year in combination with GH. Sperm counts and quality at approximately 18 years of age were not different from sperm counts and quality in controls, or from those of boys who received GH only [38].

## Conclusions

At present, accumulated evidence suggests that treatment of adolescent boys with a potent aromatase inhibitor delays bone maturation and increases predicted adult height. In contrast to gonadotropin-releasing hormone analogs, they allow the progression of physical signs of puberty, improve growth velocity, have less effect on bone mass accrual and favorably influence body composition. Based on very limited near-final height and final adult height data, they may increase final adult height, but this needs further study. The right timing and duration of the treatment are unclear, but available evidence suggests that continuation of the treatment until later stages of puberty may be needed to maintain the treatment effect. It is also unclear which compound, letrozole or anastrozole, is better in growth indications. Anastrozole has less effect on serum

**Table 3.** Suggested follow-up during aromatase inhibitor treatment in adolescent boys

| |
|---|
| *Medical history and physical examination* |
| Signs of androgen excess |
| Height, weight and sitting height |
| Pubertal staging and testicular volume |
| Joint symptoms |
| *Laboratory investigations* |
| Luteinizing hormone, follicle-stimulating hormone, testosterone, estradiol (by mass spectrometry), inhibin B |
| Alanine transaminase |
| Lipid profile |
| Blood count |
| 25-OH vitamin D |
| *Imaging studies* |
| Bone age |
| BMD (DXA) |
| Vertebral morphology by radiography (lateral projection) |
| Peripheral quantitative CT (if available) |

testosterone, which may be advantageous. Letrozole and anastrozole are generally well tolerated, but several safety issues remain inadequately studied. In particular, prospective evaluation of vertebral morphology and bone structure and density in different bone compartments needs to be done. In addition, the effect of treatment on behavior has not been evaluated in a structured manner. Aromatase inhibitor treatment is not recommended during prepuberty in growth indications. Until more long-term safety and efficacy data are available, aromatase inhibitors should be considered experimental in growth indications. However, if the use of aromatase inhibitors is considered in an individual case, adequate monitoring during the therapy is necessary (table 3).

## Disclosure Statement

The author has nothing to disclose.

## References

1 Bulun SE, Takayama K, Suzuki T, Sasano H, Yilmaz B, Sebastian S: Organization of the human aromatase P450 *(CYP19)* gene. Semin Reprod Med 2004; 22:5–9.

2 Smith EP, Boyd J, Frank GR, Takahashi H, Cohen RM, Specker B, Williams TC, Lubahn DB, Korach KS: Estrogen resistance caused by a mutation in the estrogen-receptor gene in a man. N Engl J Med 1994; 331:1056–1161.

3 Morishima A, Grumbach MM, Simpson ER, Fisher C, Qin K: Aromatase deficiency in male and female siblings caused by a novel mutation and the physiological role of estrogens. J Clin Endocrinol Metab 1995;80:3689–3398.

4 Carani C, Qin K, Simoni M, Faustini-Fustini M, Serpente S, Boyd J, Korach KS, Simpson ER: Effect of testosterone and estradiol in a man with aromatase deficiency. N Engl J Med 1997;337:91–95.

5 Wit JM, Hero M, Nunez SB: Aromatase inhibitors in pediatrics. Nat Rev Endocrinol 2011;8:135–147.
6 Leschek EW, Jones J, Barnes KM, Hill SC, Cutler GB Jr: Six-year results of spironolactone and testolactone treatment of familial male-limited precocious puberty with addition of deslorelin after central puberty onset. J Clin Endocrinol Metab 1999;84:175–118.
7 Reiter EO, Mauras N, McCormick K, Kulshreshtha B, Amrhein J, De Luca F, O'Brien S, Armstrong J, Melezinkova H: Bicalutamide plus anastrozole for the treatment of gonadotropin-independent precocious puberty in boys with testotoxicosis: a phase II, open-label pilot study (BATT). J Pediatr Endocrinol Metab 2010;23:999–1009.
8 Binder G, Iliev DI, Dufke A, Wabitsch M, Schweizer R, Ranke MB, Schmidt M: Dominant transmission of prepubertal gynecomastia due to serum estrone excess: hormonal, biochemical, and genetic analysis in a large kindred. J Clin Endocrinol Metab 2005;90: 484–492.
9 Lefevre H, Bouvattier C, Lahlou N, Adamsbaum C, Bougneres P, Carel JC: Prepubertal gynecomastia in Peutz-Jeghers syndrome: incomplete penetrance in a familial case and management with an aromatase inhibitor. Eur J Endocrinol 2006;154:221–227.
10 Grandone A, del Giudice EM, Cirillo G, Santarpia M, Coppola F, Perrone L: Prepubertal gynecomastia in two monozygotic twins with Peutz-Jeghers syndrome: two years' treatment with anastrozole and genetic study. Horm Res Paediatr 2011;75:374–379.
11 Feuillan P, Calis K, Hill S, Shawker T, Robey PG, Collins MT: Letrozole treatment of precocious puberty in girls with the McCune-Albright syndrome: a pilot study. J Clin Endocrinol Metab 2007;92:2100–2106.
12 Mieszczak J, Lowe ES, Plourde P, Eugster EA: The aromatase inhibitor anastrozole is ineffective in the treatment of precocious puberty in girls with McCune-Albright syndrome. J Clin Endocrinol Metab 2008;93:2751–2754.
13 Plourde PV, Reiter EO, Jou HC, Desrochers PE, Rubin SD, Bercu BB, Diamond FB Jr, Backeljauw PF: Safety and efficacy of anastrozole for the treatment of pubertal gynecomastia: a randomized, double-blind, placebo-controlled trial. J Clin Endocrinol Metab 2004;89:4428–4433.
14 Merke DP, Keil MF, Jones JV, Fields J, Hill S, Cutler GB Jr: Flutamide, testolactone, and reduced hydrocortisone dose maintain normal growth velocity and bone maturation despite elevated androgen levels in children with congenital adrenal hyperplasia. J Clin Endocrinol Metab 2000;85:1114–1120.
15 Santen RJ, Brodie H, Simpson ER, Siiteri PK, Brodie A: History of aromatase: saga of an important biological mediator and therapeutic target. Endocr Rev 2009;30:343–375.
16 Mauras N, O'Brien KO, Klein KO, Hayes V: Estrogen suppression in males: metabolic effects. J Clin Endocrinol Metab 2009;85:2370–2237.
17 Neely EK, Kumar RB, Payne SL, Ranadive SA, Suchet DI: Letrozole vs anastrozole for height augmentation in short pubertal males: first year data. J Clin Endocrinol Metab 2014;99:4086–4093.
18 Hero M, Norjavaara E, Dunkel L: Inhibition of estrogen biosynthesis with a potent aromatase inhibitor increases predicted adult height in boys with idiopathic short stature: a randomized controlled trial. J Clin Endocrinol Metab 2005;90:6396–6402.
19 Wickman S, Sipila I, Ankarberg-Lindgren C, Norjavaara E, Dunkel L: A specific aromatase inhibitor and potential increase in adult height in boys with delayed puberty: a randomised controlled trial. Lancet 2001;357:1743–1178.
20 Salehpour S, Alipour P, Razzaghy-Azar M, Ardeshirpour L, Shamshiri A, Monfared MF, Gharib A: A double-blind, placebo-controlled comparison of letrozole to oxandrolone effects upon growth and puberty of children with constitutional delay of puberty and idiopathic short stature. Horm Res Paediatr 2010;74:428–435.
21 Mauras N, Gonzalez de Pijem L, Hsiang HY, Desrosiers P, Rapaport R, Schwartz ID, Klein KO, Singh RJ, Miyamoto A, Bishop K: Anastrozole increases predicted adult height of short adolescent males treated with growth hormone: a randomized, placebo-controlled, multicenter trial for one to three years. J Clin Endocrinol Metab 2008;93:823–831.
22 Wickman S, Dunkel L: Inhibition of P450 aromatase enhances gonadotropin secretion in early and midpubertal boys: evidence for a pituitary site of action of endogenous E. J Clin Endocrinol Metab 2001;86: 4887–4894.
23 Hero M, Wickman S, Hanhijarvi R, Siimes MA, Dunkel L: Pubertal upregulation of erythropoiesis in boys is determined primarily by androgen. J Pediatr 2005;146:245–252.
24 Hero M, Wickman S, Dunkel L: Treatment with the aromatase inhibitor letrozole during adolescence increases near-final height in boys with constitutional delay of puberty. Clin Endocrinol (Oxf) 2006;64: 510–513.
25 Hero M, Toiviainen-Salo S, Wickman S, Makitie O, Dunkel L: Vertebral morphology in aromatase inhibitor-treated males with idiopathic short stature or constitutional delay of puberty. J Bone Miner Res 2010;25:1536–1543.
26 Taxel P, Kennedy DG, Fall PM, Willard AK, Clive JM, Raisz LG: The effect of aromatase inhibition on sex steroids, gonadotropins, and markers of bone turnover in older men. J Clin Endocrinol Metab 2001;86:2869–2874.

27 Hero M, Makitie O, Kroger H, Nousiainen E, Toivi-ainen-Salo S, Dunkel L: Impact of aromatase inhibitor therapy on bone turnover, cortical bone growth and vertebral morphology in pre- and peripubertal boys with idiopathic short stature. Horm Res 2009; 71:290–297.
28 Wickman S, Saukkonen T, Dunkel L: The role of sex steroids in the regulation of insulin sensitivity and serum lipid concentrations during male puberty: a prospective study with a P450-aromatase inhibitor. Eur J Endocrinol 2002;146:339–346.
29 Hero M, Ankarberg-Lindgren C, Taskinen MR, Dunkel L: Blockade of oestrogen biosynthesis in peripubertal boys: effects on lipid metabolism, insulin sensitivity, and body composition. Eur J Endocrinol 2006;155:453–460.
30 Kampen DL, Sherwin BB: Estrogen use and verbal memory in healthy postmenopausal women. Obstet Gynecol 1994;83:979–983.
31 Cherrier MM, Matsumoto AM, Amory JK, Ahmed S, Bremner W, Peskind ER, Raskind MA, Johnson M, Craft S: The role of aromatization in testosterone supplementation: effects on cognition in older men. Neurology 2005;64:290–296.
32 Hero M, Maury S, Luotoniemi E, Service E, Dunkel L: Cognitive effects of aromatase inhibitor therapy in peripubertal boys. Eur J Endocrinol 2010;163:149–155.
33 Oz OK, Hirasawa G, Lawson J, Nanu L, Constantinescu A, Antich PP, Mason RP, Tsyganov E, Parkey RW, Zerwekh JE, Simpson ER: Bone phenotype of the aromatase deficient mouse. J Steroid Biochem Mol Biol 2001;79:49–59.
34 Shetty G, Krishnamurthy H, Krishnamurthy HN, Bhatnagar S, Moudgal RN: Effect of estrogen deprivation on the reproductive physiology of male and female primates. J Steroid Biochem Mol Biol 1997; 61:157–166.
35 Aquila S, Sisci D, Gentile M, Carpino A, Middea E, Catalano S, Rago V, Ando S: Towards a physiological role for cytochrome P450 aromatase in ejaculated human sperm. Hum Reprod 2003;18:1650–1659.
36 Raman JD, Schlegel PN: Aromatase inhibitors for male infertility. J Urol 2002;167(2 pt 1):624–629.
37 Ramasamy R, Ricci JA, Palermo GD, Gosden LV, Rosenwaks Z, Schlegel PN: Successful fertility treatment for Klinefelter's syndrome. J Urol 2009;182: 1108–1113.
38 Mauras N, Bell J, Snow BG, Winslow KL: Sperm analysis in growth hormone-deficient adolescents previously treated with an aromatase inhibitor: comparison with normal controls. Fertil Steril 2005;84: 239–242.
39 Geffner ME: Aromatase inhibitors to augment height: continued caution and study required. J Clin Res Pediatr Endocrinol. 2009;1:256–261.

Matti Hero, MD, PhD
Children's Hospital
Helsinki University Central Hospital (HUCH)
PO Box 705, FI-00029 HUS, Helsinki (Finland)
E-Mail matti.hero@hus.fi

Cappa M, Cianfarani S, Ghizzoni L, Loche S, Maghnie M (eds): Advanced Therapies in Pediatric Endocrinology and Diabetology. Endocr Dev. Basel, Karger, 2016, vol 30, pp 141–146 (DOI: 10.1159/000439339)

# Gene Therapy for Rare Central Nervous System Diseases Comes to Age

Patrick Aubourg

INSERM U1169, Department of Pediatric Neurology, Bicêtre Hospital, and Paris-Sud University, Le Kremlin-Bicêtre, France

**Abstract**

Gene therapy for rare inherited neurologic diseases has entered the clinics. One strategy relies upon the replacement of brain microglia using hematopoietic stem cell gene therapy with lentiviral vectors. Therapeutic success using this approach has been obtained in X-linked adrenoleukodystrophy and metachromatic leukodystrophy. The other strategy relies upon the intracerebral administration of adeno-associated virus vectors encoding lysosomal enzymes. Therapeutic trials are ongoing in Batten's disease, metachromatic leukodystrophy, and Sanfilippo type A and B diseases.



The central nervous system (CNS) is a complex organ with intricate and complex interconnections between various types of neurons, glia and other cells. At first glance, the CNS seems to be a complicated target for gene-therapeutic interventions. With significant advances in technologies, the use of viral vectors to deliver genes to the nervous system has however come of age and is starting to show promise in the treatment of selected CNS disorders. Two different strategies have been developed and have entered the clinics: hematopoietic stem cell (HSC) gene therapy with lentiviral vectors (LV) and direct intracerebral gene therapy with adeno-associated virus (AAV) vectors.

## Hematopoietic Stem Cell Gene Therapy

The advantages of cell vehicles for virus delivery include the ability to carry out genetic correction of cells ex vivo, where conditions can be optimized and cells selected for specific properties, gene expression and safety. Transduced cell types envisaged for this purpose in the brain include astrocytes, neural precursor cells and HSCs. Since the first attempt to perform allogeneic HSC transplantation ('bone marrow transplantation') in Hurler's disease, it is known that following transplant, bone marrow-derived cells can enter the brain and give rise to a subset of glial cells called microglia that share the same origin as macrophages and monocytes. A major advance in the field of gene therapy was the demonstration that safe LVs (i.e. those unable to replicate) derived from human immunodeficiency virus could infect dividing as well as nondividing cells, including HSCs [1]. LVs have a packaging capacity of approximately 8 kb and are usually generated (pseudo-typed) with the G-glycoprotein envelope from vesicular stomatitis virus. Owing to their property to integrate definitively the transgene into the host cell genome, they allow long-term transgene expression in HSCs that divide and give rise to red blood cells, T and B lymphocytes, and myelomonocytic cells including microglial precursors. One good example of the use of HSC transplantation with LV is cerebral X-linked adrenoleukodystrophy [2]. In this paradigm, autologous HSC transplantation is performed, but cells are genetically corrected ex vivo prior to injection into the patient after myeloablation. Following engraftment, microglial precursors enter the blood circulation, cross the blood-brain barrier and then differentiate into microglial cells expressing the *ABCD1* gene. HSC gene therapy with LV has been performed in 4 boys with cerebral X-linked adrenoleukodystrophy at early-stage cerebral demyelination. Like allogeneic HSC transplantation, it allowed to arrest definitively the progression of cerebral demyelination in the 4 treated patients with good to very good quality of life in 3 of them. In terms of clinical benefits, HSC gene therapy with LV was not superior to allogeneic HSC transplantation but had the great advantage to overcome the need for an HLA-matched donor and not be associated with the risk of graft failure and severe graft-versus-host disease, which occur each in approximately 15% of allogeneic HSC transplantations and result very often in the death of the treated patients. The same strategy has been used to treat metachromatic leukodystrophy (MLD) patients at a presymptomatic stage [3]. In this paradigm, HSC are engineered to overexpress the arylsulfatase A (ARSA) lysosomal enzyme in order to achieve higher expression of ARSA in brain microglia than after conventional allogeneic HSC transplantation [4]. Since the ARSA enzyme can be secreted by corrected cells and recaptured by noncorrected cells, the spectrum of enzymatically corrected cells may involve other cells than microglia (neurons, oligodendrocytes or astrocytes). This is in sharp contrast with X-linked adrenoleukodystrophy since the peroxisomal membrane transporter encoded by the *ABCD1* gene cannot be secreted. One major limitation of HSC gene therapy is however the time (14–16 months) required in order to achieve a sufficient number of corrected microglia in the brain to obtain a therapeutic effect, i.e. to arrest neurodegeneration. This explains the failure of this approach in cerebral X-linked adrenoleukodystrophy at an advanced stage of cerebral demyelination when the disease progresses rapidly and in symptomatic MLD with cerebral demyelination and rapidly progressive disease. The integration of LV into the genome may potentially result in genotoxicity, i.e. conferring an abnormal growth rate (due to activation of oncogenes following the nearby insertion of LV vector) to corrected hematopoietic cells that may end up ultimately in leukemia. Such adverse events have however not been observed in X-linked adrenoleukodystrophy and MLD patients up to now during a follow-up of 8 years. HSC gene therapy with LV is now envisaged to treat Hurler's disease and Krabbe's disease, two other lysosomal CNS diseases. In Krabbe's disease however, the very rapid progression of neurodegeneration in patients with the infantile form of the disease is likely to preclude any therapeutic effect in due time that could result in a good quality of life in treated patients. Therefore, a combination of HSC gene therapy with intracerebral gene therapy may be beneficial in this disease.

### Brain Gene Therapy with Adeno-Associated Virus Vectors

Many viral vectors are used in preclinical research for brain gene therapy, and the vectorology methodologies are continually undergoing refinement. Today, the most common gene therapy with viral vectors in use for clinical application in rare CNS diseases remain AAVs owing to their safety profile and relatively simple manufacturing process. AAVs are simple capsid virions – a nucleic acid genome encased in a proteinaceous shell called capsid. The efficiency of AAV vectors to transduce a specific cell population in the CNS, called *tropism,* depends on their capacity to bind receptors at the cell surface specific to each AAV serotype. The density of these receptors varies among different types of neuronal cells and the identity of these receptors has not been identified for most AAV vectors, which precludes the possibility to choose a particular AAV serotype to target a specific neuronal cell type. As there are species differences in AAV tropism, the issue has to be addressed at best in nonhuman primates with the hypothesis that AAV tropism in this species should be similar to AAV tropism in humans. Following binding at the cell surface, capsid virions undergo receptor-mediated endocytosis, and as the endosomal compartment acidifies, the capsid breaks down. The viral genome containing the therapeutic gene, which has to be modified to avoid infectious replication of viral particles, is then released into the cytoplasm and transported to the nucleus. Once in the nucleus, the viral genome remains in a single- or double-strand DNA episomal form without the capacity to integrate into the genome like retroviruses or LVs. One main limitation of AAV vectors is their small capacity (4.5 kb) of transgene size. The choice of a promoter to drive optimal transgene expression in specific cell populations may be crucial because housekeeping or ubiquitous promoters (artificial promoters made of a mix of viral and human sequences) do not allow to express transgenes at the same levels in all types of neuronal cells. In addition, there is no possibility to drive physiological expression of therapeutic transgenes (even with the use of cell-specific promoters) and only a low/medium/high level of transgene expression can be achieved according to the promoter to be used. Potential toxicity due to overexpression of a therapeutic transgene must therefore be assessed in preclinical steps. Of note also, the expression of the therapeutic transgene cannot be even in all corrected neuronal cells. This is due to the fact that cells may contain variable copy numbers of episomal forms of therapeutic transgenes, which may result in variable transgene expression. The maximum expression of transgenes is obtained at the injection site where transduced cells contain the highest copy number of the transgenes. AAV vectors have also the capacity to be transported to some extent anterogradely or retrogradely along axons, which may increase the expression of the therapeutic gene distant from the injection site [5]. Each AAV serotype has advantages and drawbacks. AAV5, AAV9 and AAVrh10 seem to diffuse more widely than AAV2 from injection sites in the brain, and AAV4 primarily transduces ependymal cells. In the cerebellum, AAV5 transduces Purkinje cells but not granule cells. Retrograde transport of AAV9 is more efficient than that of AAV2 [6]; recently, AAV9 was shown to cross the blood-brain barrier after intravenous injection and infect astrocytes or neurons of the brain and spinal cord [7, 8]. Most of these results have however been obtained in mice and must be reassessed in non-human primates using the same research grade quality of vectors, in particular in terms of the therapeutic index. Eighty percent of the human population is positive for antibodies to AAV serotype 2, with 30–70% of those individuals having neutralizing antibodies as well. Preexisting immunity to any AAV serotypes may result in a significant reduction in neuronal cell transduction. At least 20–30% of the human population have also neutralizing antibodies against AAV9 and AAVrh10 vectors despite the fact these AAV vectors have been isolated from monkeys. Although the CNS is considered as immunoprivileged, one should not underestimate the risk of immune reactions against the therapeutic transgene. In patients with a null mutation of the disease gene resulting in the complete absence of the encoded protein, a T-cell reaction against the therapeutic protein encoded by the AAV vector and produced by the transduced cells may result in their destruction and a neuroinflammatory disease. One main limitation of brain gene therapy with AAV vectors is the limited diffusion of viral capsids from the injection sites. This implicates that multiple brain injections must be performed to achieve reasonable expression of the therapeutic transgene throughout the brain. The risk of hematoma following brain biopsy is approximately 3%. The more injections are performed within the brain, the higher the risk of hematoma with the ensuing serious adverse effects. On the other hand, when the protein encoded by the therapeutic transgene can be secreted and recaptured at distant sites by other cells (like lysosomal enzymes), this may enhance the efficiency of the therapeutic procedure. Little attention has been paid up to now on how to deliver viral vectors within the CNS (brain or spinal cord through intrathecal delivery). This includes not only the devices for injection, but also the volume in which the viral vector is diluted and the rate of injection. Intensive work is clearly needed to optimize vector delivery within the CNS. Despite the high transduction efficiency of AAV for neurons, their tropism frequently does not match the therapeutic need. In particular, these vectors have no or little tropism for oligodendrocytes and infect astrocytes with little efficacy. Several strategies have been envisaged to engineer viral vectors to a specific cell type [9]. One is 'pseudotyping' which involves transferring viral attachment proteins within a family of AAV vectors. Pseudotyping is however limited by the number of viral attachment proteins for which receptors are expressed exclusively and abundantly on the target cells of interest. Another strategy is 'vector targeting' using adaptors. The use of adaptor proteins can be applied even with a limited knowledge of the viral structure. Adaptors are molecules with dual specificities: one end binds the viral attachment protein and the other binds the receptor on the target cell. The advantages of this approach are its great flexibility, as different adaptors can readily be coupled to the same vector, and the fact that it does not require changes in the vector structure that could be detrimental to vector production or gene transfer. One major disadvantage of the adaptors relates to the potentially suboptimal stability of the vector-adaptor complex, especially in vivo, which might result from unforeseen interactions with factors that perturb the noncovalent binding. The last one is 'genetic incorporation of targeting ligands'. Genetic fusion of ligands into the capsid or the envelope protein yields a single virion molecule that recognizes the target cell. This has driven library selection approaches, which aim to display the ligand in the context of the viral attachment protein and then select for the desired increase in infectivity by binding to a column that displays the targeting receptor; this is certainly one of the most promising approaches. Screening a phage library in vivo by panning to identify peptides that bind the vascular endothelia in the brain has allowed to expand the biodistribution of intravenously injected AAV from the liver as a predominant target to the CNS, and to treat with success a mouse model of lysosomal storage disease [10].

The proof of concept of AAV brain gene therapy has been demonstrated in many animal models of rare CNS diseases. They include in particular mouse, dog or cat models of mucopolysaccharidosis (MPS) VII (ß-glucuronidase deficiency), MPS I (Hurler's disease), MPS IIIB (α-L-iduronidase deficiency), MPS IIB (Sanfilippo type B, α-N-acetylglucosaminidase deficiency), Niemann-Pick type A disease (acid sphingomyelinase deficiency), Krabbe's disease (galactocerebrosidase deficiency), MLD (ARSA deficiency), Batten's disease (palmitoyl protein thioesterase-1 and tripeptidyl peptidase I deficiency) and α-mannosidosis. A gene therapy trial has already been performed some years ago in Batten's disease with AAV2 vector [11] and new trials with more efficacious AAV vectors are ongoing in MLD, Batten's disease and Sanfilippo type A and B diseases (see clinicaltrials.gov).

## References


1 Naldini L, Blömer U, Gallay P, Ory D, Mulligan R, Gage FH, Verma IM, Trono D: In vivo gene delivery and stable transduction of nondividing cells by a lentiviral vector. Science 1996;272:263–267.

2 Cartier N, Hacein-Bey-Abina S, Bartholomae CC, Veres G, Schmidt M, Kutschera I, Vidaud M, Abel U, Dal-Cortivo L, Caccavelli L, Mahlaoui N, Kiermer V, Mittelstaedt D, Bellesme C, Lahlou N, Lefrère F, Blanche S, Audit M, Payen E, Leboulch P, l'Homme B, Bougnères P, Von Kalle C, Fischer A, Cavazzana-Calvo M, Aubourg P: Hematopoietic stem cell gene therapy with a lentiviral vector in X-linked adrenoleukodystrophy. Science 2009;326:818–812.

3 Biffi A, Montini E, Lorioli L, Cesani M, Fumagalli F, Plati T, Baldoli C, Martino S, Calabria A, Canale S, Benedicenti F, Vallanti G, Biasco L, Leo S, Kabbara N, Zanetti G, Rizzo WB, Mehta NA, Cicalese MP, Casiraghi M, Boelens JJ, Del Carro U, Dow DJ, Schmidt M, Assanelli A, Neduva V, Di Serio C, Stupka E, Gardner J, von Kalle C, Bordignon C, Ciceri F, Rovelli A, Roncarolo MG, Aiuti A, Sessa M, Naldini L: Lentiviral hematopoietic stem cell gene therapy benefits metachromatic leukodystrophy. Science 2013;341:1233158.

4 Biffi A, Capotondo A, Fasano S, del Carro U, Marchesini S, Azuma H, Malaguti MC, Amadio S, Brambilla R, Grompe M, Bordignon C, Quattrini A, Naldini L: Gene therapy of metachromatic leukodystrophy reverses neurological damage and deficits in mice. J Clin Invest 2006;116:3070–3082.

5 Cearley CN, Wolfe JH: A single injection of an adeno-associated virus vector into nuclei with divergent connections results in widespread vector distribution in the brain and global correction of a neurogenetic disease. J Neurosci 2007;27:9928–9940.

6 Cearley CN, Wolfe JH: Transduction characteristics of adeno-associated virus vectors expressing cap serotypes 7, 8, 9, and Rh10 in the mouse brain. Mol Ther 2006;13:528–537.

7 Foust KD, Nurre E, Montgomery CL, Hernandez A, Chan CM, Kaspar BK: Intravascular AAV9 preferentially targets neonatal neurons and adult astrocytes. Nat Biotechnol 2009;27:59–65.

8 Duque S, Joussemet B, Riviere C, Marais T, Dubreil L, Douar AM, Fyfe J, Moullier P, Colle MA, Barkats M: Intravenous administration of self-complementary AAV9 enables transgene delivery to adult motor neurons. Mol Ther 2009;17:1187–1196.

9 Waehler R, Russel SJ, Curiel DT: Engineering targeted viral vectors for gene therapy. Nat Rev Genet 2007;8:573–587.

10 Chen YH, Chang M, Davidson BL: Molecular signatures of disease brain endothelia provide new sites for CNS-directed enzyme therapy. Nat Med 2009;15: 1215–1218.

11 Worgall S, Sondhi D, Hackett NR, Kosofsky B, Kekatpure MV, Neyzi N, Dyke JP, Ballon D, Heier L, Greenwald BM, Christos P, Mazumdar M, Souweidane MM, Kaplitt MG, Crystal RG: Treatment of late infantile neuronal ceroid lipofuscinosis by CNS administration of a serotype 2 adeno-associated virus expressing CLN2 cDNA. Hum Gene Ther 2008;19: 463–474.



Patrick Aubourg, MD
INSERM U1169, Department of Pediatric Neurology
Bicêtre Hospital, and Paris-Sud University
80 rue du Général Leclerc, FR–94270 Le Kremlin-Bicêtre (France)
E-Mail patrick.aubourg@inserm.fr

Cappa M, Cianfarani S, Ghizzoni L, Loche S, Maghnie M (eds): Advanced Therapies in Pediatric Endocrinology and Diabetology. Endocr Dev. Basel, Karger, 2016, vol 30, pp 147–160 (DOI: 10.1159/000439340)

# Novel Therapeutic Targets and Drug Candidates for Modifying Disease Progression in Adrenoleukodystrophy

Aurora Pujol

Laboratory of Neurometabolic Diseases and Pathologic Anatomy Service, Institute of Neuropathology, Bellvitge Biomedical Research Institute (IDIBELL)-Hospital Universitari de Bellvitge, L'Hospitalet de Llobregat and Center for Biomedical Research on Rare Diseases (CIBERER), U759, ISCIII, and Catalan Institution of Research and Advanced Studies (ICREA), Barcelona, Spain

**Abstract**

X-linked adrenoleukodystrophy (X-ALD) is the most frequent inherited monogenic demyelinating disease. It is often lethal and currently lacks a satisfactory therapy. The disease is caused by loss of function of the *ABCD1* gene, a peroxisomal ATP-binding cassette transporter, resulting in the accumulation of very-long-chain fatty acids (VLCFA) in organs and plasma. Recent findings on pathomechanisms of the peroxisomal neurometabolic disease X-ALD have provided important clues on therapeutic targets. Here we describe the impact of chronic redox imbalance caused by the excess VLCFA on mitochondrial biogenesis and respiration, and explore the consequences on the protein quality control systems essential for cell survival, such as the proteasome and autophagic flux. Defective proteostasis, together with mitochondrial malfunction, is a hallmark of the most prevalent neurodegenerative diseases, including Alzheimer's disease and Parkinson's disease, and of the aging process. Thus, we discuss molecular targets and emerging treatment options that may be common to both multifactorial neurodegenerative disorders and X-ALD. New-generation antioxidants, some of them mitochondrial targeted, mitochondrial biogenesis boosters such as pioglitazone and resveratrol, and the mTOR inhibitor temsirolimus hold promise as disease-modifying therapies.



## X-Linked Adrenoleukodystrophy: The Disease

X-linked adrenoleukodystrophy (X-ALD; OMIM No. 300100) is the most common peroxisomal disorder and monogenic leukodystrophy. Patients suffer from adrenal insufficiency, central inflammatory demyelination in the brain and/or slowly progressing axonal degeneration of the corticospinal tracts, resulting in spastic paraparesis [1–3]. X-ALD is caused by mutations in the *ABCD1* gene (Xq28), which encodes the ATP-binding cassette transporter, an integral peroxisomal membrane protein.

The ABCD1 protein imports very-long-chain fatty acids (VLCFA) and VLCFA-CoA esters into the peroxisome for degradation [4, 5]. The defective function of the ABCD1 transporter leads to VLCFA excess due to decreased β-oxidation of these fatty acids in peroxisomes [5, 6], leading to a disturbed fatty acid profile in tissues and plasma, particularly involving hexacosanoic acid (C26:0) and C26:0-containing lipids. These are used as pathognomonic markers for the biochemical diagnosis of X-ALD [7, 8].

Despite being a single-gene disease, X-ALD is a complex inherited syndrome in which the same mutation in the *ABCD1* gene can lead clinically to very distinct phenotypes [1–3, 9]. Loss-of-function mutations in this protein are the cause of the disease, which is characterized by three main distinct phenotypes. Cerebral childhood ALD (cALD), which affects boys between 5 and 12 years of age, manifests in ~35% of all X-ALD patients and exhibits strong inflammatory demyelination with autoimmune components, leading to death within few years. Adrenomyeloneuropathy (AMN) is the most frequent manifestation of X-ALD and affects adult patients. AMN patients present peripheral neuropathy and distal axonopathy involving corticospinal tracts of the spinal cord – but neither brain neuroinflammation nor major demyelination – with spastic paraparesis as major symptoms. Intermediate forms with noninflammatory childhood cerebral demyelination occur, as do mixed forms, with around 20% of all AMN patients developing a cerebral inflammatory disease at later stages than in cALD. X-ALD is the most common genetic cause of Addison's disease. A majority of patients additionally suffer from adrenal insufficiency (65% of AMN and 85% of cALD patients), which affects the glucocorticoid and later the mineralocorticoid functions. Onset of acute adrenal insufficiency may occur between 5 and 35 years of age, and it can remain the only clinical expression of X-ALD for decades [1–3, 9, 10]. Interestingly, all clinical phenotypes can occur within the same family, indicating that there is no direct phenotype-genotype correlation [1–3, 9]. Female carriers frequently develop AMN, with symptoms such as myelopathy and peripheral neuropathy [11].

To date, the only treatment is allogeneic bone marrow transplantation, which is associated with a high morbidity and mortality, and is available only to nearly asymptomatic X-ALD children [12]. This alternative treatment has the same indications as bone marrow transplantation, meaning that it can be applied only to a small subset of patients with few to no symptoms [13]. A novel gene therapy strategy uses adeno-associated virus serotype 9 to express human *ABCD1,* which has yielded promising results in a mouse model of X-ALD [14]. However, a recent report suggests that allogeneic bone marrow transplant in cALD does arrest inflammatory progression and death, but does not prevent the adult AMN phenotype from developing AMN in adulthood [15].

Thus, for AMN patients there is no satisfactory treatment to date. Oral administration of 'Lorenzo's oil' has been used, but its clinical efficacy and clinical indications have been controversial for more than 15 years [16]. Nonetheless, more recent successful pharmacological preclinical tests in the X-ALD mouse model warrant translation into the clinic [17–19, 20].

## Mouse Models of X-Linked Adrenoleukodystrophy: Limitations and Applications

The classical knockout of the murine *Abcd1* gene, the X-ALD mouse model, does not exhibit signs of demyelination in spite of the accumulation of VLCFA in the brain [21]. This mouse model shows instead a phenotype resembling late-onset axonal degeneration in spinal cords presented by most AMN patients, which is characterized by spastic paraparesis due to degeneration of corticospinal tracts, but without signs of active inflammatory demyelination in the brain. In the mouse, mainly axonal pathology is detectable in sciatic nerves and long tracts of spinal cords, but not in the brain. This is correlated with slower motor nerve conduction, and with disability signs in rotarod, treadmill, bar cross and clasping tests, of very late onset (around 20 months of age) [22–24]. Thus, the phenotype of *Abcd1*$^{-}$ mice mimics features of human AMN, providing a model for investigating disease pathogenesis. Also, this model provides evidence of axonal degeneration prior to myelin degeneration, an important finding that strongly suggests that the underlying phenotype in the human disease is AMN, with full penetrance at 50 years of age [25].

In an attempt to achieve a more severe phenotype, we generated double-mutants of *Abcd1* and its closest homolog, the *Abcd2* gene, which exhibits overlapping biochemical and physiological functions with *Abcd1* [6, 26–29], and is able to compensate for *Abcd1* loss in vivo [25]. *Abcd2* is thus a prime therapeutic target [30–33]. These double-mutant mice exhibited a more pronounced and earlier-onset axonal degenerative phenotype, manifesting at around 12 months of age and, thus, constituting the model of choice for therapeutic assays [25]. Both *Abcd1*$^{-}$ and *Abcd1*$^{-}$/*Abcd2*$^{-/-}$ mice are bona fide models of mild, late-onset axonopathy exhibited by AMN patients. These models are instrumental in dissecting pathomechanisms of AMN [34–38] and, importantly, in pinpointing therapeutic targets and evaluating novel treatments [14, 17–19, 20, 39].

In these models, an important degree of chronic neuroinflammation with astrocytosis and microgliosis is present in spinal cords of both, the *Abcd1 null* and more markedly in the double *Abcd1/Abcd2* mouse model. Interestingly, a functional genomics approach carried out on the *Abcd1 null* model has unraveled a signature characterized by oxidative stress, mitochondrial dysregulation, adipocytokine signaling and chronic inflammation routes, including NF-κB activation with production of proinflammatory cytokines detected in spinal cords and plasma [38]. These findings challenge the notion that inflammatory reactions only occur in the most severe forms of X-ALD, and provide a basis to argue that a low-grade proinflammatory reaction initiated by VLCFA may adopt a more aggressive profile should a second (or third) hit appear [40]. These additional modifier genes or epigenetic, environmental or stochastic events, which ignite a full-blown cerebral inflammatory demyelination in cALD or cerebral AMN (cAMN) patients, have not been identified as of today. Thus, a suitable animal model that serves as a tool for the development of therapeutic strategies for the lethal stages of this disorder is still missing.

### *Early Oxidative Stress and Damage*

Oxidative stress is defined as a pathological condition that results from a redox disequilibrium leading to an excess of reactive oxygen species (ROS). A consequence of ROS production is interaction with cellular biomolecules, in particular DNA, lipids and proteins, which are then modified. Proteins can be directly damaged by ROS or indirectly by reacting with active aldehyde products of lipid peroxidation, e.g. malondialdehyde or hydroxynonenal, or as a result of alterations in membrane lipid microenvironment secondary to peroxidative processes. These changes are detrimental if the modified residues are essential for the activity or turnover of the protein [41]. Moreover, oxidative lesions can also transform lipid properties and induce mutations in mitochondrial and nuclear DNA, causing mitochondrial dysfunction and pathology [42].

Taking advantage of the *Abcd1*$^-$ mouse model and keeping track of the data obtained with expression microarrays [38], we uncovered an early-onset oxidative damage, which may be a major contributor to disease pathogenesis in the mouse [18, 34, 40, 43, 44]. This is a common feature to neurodegenerative diseases and aging, and is found in X-ALD patients in brain tissue as well as in peripheral cells such as fibroblasts, erythrocytes, peripheral mononuclear cells and plasma [31, 43–46].

*Abcd1*$^-$ mice present accumulation of malonaldehyde-lysine, a consequence of lipoxidative damage to proteins, in spinal cords as early as 3.5 months of age. At 12 months, *Abcd1*$^-$ mice accumulate additional oxidative damage products arising from metal-catalyzed oxidation and glycoxidation/lipoxidation to proteins. We also detected several oxidatively modified proteins, mostly belonging to the Krebs cycle, oxidative phosphorylation (OXPHOS) and glycolysis [37, 47]. This was associated with impaired activities of pyruvate kinase, and lowered levels of ATP and NADH, as well as reduced glutathione (GSH) [47]. Finally, a wide array of mitochondrial genes related to the pyruvate and oxoglutarate dehydrogenase complexes, tricarboxylic acid cycle, OXPHOS system and antioxidant defenses were dysregulated in microarray analysis [38].

Thus, in X-ALD, we find a prime example of intertwined redox and metabolic homeostasis in the nervous system. Diminished levels of ATP have also been described in mouse models of Alzheimer's disease (AD) and Parkinson's disease (PD) [48, 49], although the ratios of NAD/NADH, which are of paramount importance, have not been systematically measured in most prevalent neurodegenerative diseases.

Importantly, we observed that a trigger of redox imbalance was the raised levels of VLCFA. Indeed, C26:0 in excess is able to generate ROS and decrease mitochondrial membrane potential and levels of reduced GSH in human X-ALD fibroblasts [34].

Similar studies showed that VLCFA was able to depolarize mitochondria and increase ROS in immortalized or primary neural cell cultures [50–53].

Next, we found that a combination of antioxidants carefully selected on the basis of their intrinsic properties, N-acetylcysteine, α-lipoic acid and vitamin E, showed synergistic effects in vitro. N-acetylcysteine is a replenisher of GSH, and vitamin E is a lipophilic compound that penetrates cellular membranes (including mitochondria) and prevents the PUFA lateral chains of complex lipids to oxidize, thus halting an oxidative chain reaction most likely damaging membranes. Lipoic acid is of particular interest as it is at the same time a scavenger of ROS [54] and a cofactor of the Krebs cycle enzyme α-ketoglutarate dehydrogenase and other enzymes which are oxidized in X-ALD. Lately, lipoic acid has been shown to rescue the hypometabolic state in a mouse model of AD characterized by low levels of glutamine, glutamate, aspartate and N-acetylaspartate, i.e. metabolites of the tricarboxylic acid cycle [55]. We thus treated the X-ALD mice with the cocktail mentioned above, and observed neutralized oxidative stress and lesions to proteins; preserved bioenergetic homeostasis by recovering normal levels of oxidation on key proteins of the Krebs cycle and glycolysis; halted immunohistological signs of axonal degeneration, and decreased locomotor impairment in bar cross and treadmill tests [18, 47].

These results provide conceptual proof of C26:0-induced oxidative stress as a major causative disease-driving factor in X-ALD, thus warranting translation into clinical trials for AMN patients and inviting assessment of antioxidant strategies in other diseases with axonal degeneration in which oxidative damage may play a role.

### *Effect of Excess C26:0 on Mitochondria*

A deficient redox homeostasis linked to mitochondrial dysfunction is key to axonal degeneration in several neurodegenerative diseases [56, 57]. Mitochondria are both very sensitive to oxidative damage and the main source of ROS, in particular when the mitochondrial electron transport chain (ETC) is malfunctioning. Therefore, the accumulation of damaged mitochondria usually correlates with disease progression [56, 58]. In axons, mitochondria provide a substantial part of the energy required during neurotransmission, and their transport to ATP-demanding areas is tightly regulated. Nonetheless, axonal mitochondria are more vulnerable than their cellular counterparts, as the mitochondria with their elongated shape require to fit with the axon morphology, and are more reliant on fusion-fission events to exchange material among them. An imbalance in the triad ROS/ATP/calcium that overcomes the homeostatic capacity of the mitochondria initiates a toxic cycle of events that will ultimately activate the axonal degeneration program. For instance, mitochondrial ROS may oxidize and inhibit the OXPHOS system, inducing a decline in the ATP production. This energetic failure, in turn, impairs the ATP-dependent ionic pumps, triggering a massive calcium influx. Furthermore, ROS do not only impair the OXPHOS system but also promote the opening of the mitochondrial permeability transition pore (mPTP) leading to a subsequent efflux of calcium from the mitochondria to the cytosol. Calcium overload in the cytoplasm triggers then calcium-dependent activation of calpains. These proteases disassemble the microtubule structure and impair the correct transport along the axon. All these events will result in axonal swelling, loss of axonal continuity and, eventually, axonal destruction [59].

In X-ALD, a very similar scenario takes place with unbalanced ROS/ATP/$Ca^{2+}$ homeostasis. Mitochondria appear to be the main source of ROS in X-ALD fibroblasts when cells are exposed to an excess of C26:0, as determined through measuring intramitochondrial ROS by MitoSOX or by using mitochondrial uncouplers. Excess of C26:0 also inhibits OXPHOS in fibroblasts [37]. Defective OXPHOS was also observed in both 158N oligodendrocytes and SK-NB-E neuronal cells when exposed to VLCFA excess [50, 53] and in isolated brain mitochondria, which increase ROS production and diminish $Ca^{2+}$ uptake capacity [60]. However, a systematic assessment of additional cellular sources of ROS in X-ALD (peroxisomes, xanthine oxidase and NADPH oxidases) in relevant models of the disease, such as primary cultures of neural cells or, ideally, in vivo in the mouse nervous system, is warranted.

The molecular mechanisms by which the VLCFA excess triggers oxidative stress in mitochondria in X-ALD is far from clear. We hypothesize that excess C26:0 could alter the permeability of the inner mitochondrial membrane by replacing the lateral chains of phospholipid bilayers and physically interfering with the assembly of OXPHOS system, or by increasing membrane microviscosity [61] and provoking its disruption [62]. This could elicit electron leakage, promoting ROS generation from the ETC. In the same manner, mitochondrial inner membrane instability could allow the proton flux into the matrix, decreasing mitochondrial inner membrane potential and possibly triggering OXPHOS dysfunction. Indeed, we revealed defective respiration under uncoupled conditions both in X-ALD fibroblasts and in *Abcd1*$^{-}$ spinal cords, suggesting a specific impairment of the activity of complex V/$H^{+}$-ATP synthase, which correlates with the oxidation of several subunits of complex V and III of OXPHOS [37].

Recent advances in the study of the mPTP indicate that dimeric ATP synthase is a bona fide component of the mPTP and interacts with the gate opener cyclophilin D (CypD) [63]. We have provided evidence of impaired mitochondrial metabolism in X-ALD fibroblasts, which cannot survive when forced to rely on mitochondrial energy production, i.e. on incubation in galactose [20, 36, 37]. Oxidative stress induced under galactose conditions leads to mitochondrial damage in the form of mitochondrial inner membrane potential dissipation, ATP drop and necrotic cell death, together with increased expression of and oxidative modifications in the CypD protein [36]. Thereby, we posit that in X-ALD, mPTP formation is favored by the increased amounts of oxidized CypD and complex V/$H^{+}$-ATP synthase. Interestingly, inhibition of CypD genetically or pharmacologically with cyclosporine A prevents mitochondrial dysfunction in many age-related neurodegenerative disease models such as

AD, PD, amyotrophic lateral sclerosis (ALS) and multiple sclerosis, indicating that CypD is a prime therapeutic target for these disorders [64, 65]. Notably, treatment with antioxidants normalizes the markers of mitochondrial damage in fibroblasts from X-ALD patients, including CypD oxidative modifications, and has reversed CypD induction in other neurodegenerative disorders in vitro and in vivo [36, 37, 64]. These findings provide mechanistic insight into the beneficial effects of antioxidants in neurodegenerative and nonneurodegenerative CypD-dependent disorders. All in all, these evidences are sufficient to propose inclusion of X-ALD in a growing number of secondary mitochondriopathies [66]. It follows that mitochondrial-targeted antioxidants may be indicated in this disorder. Indeed, a phase II clinical trial with the antioxidant EPI-743 for AMN patients is planned [Bertini E., pers. commun.]. EPI-743 is a *p*-benzoquinone analog that is 1,000 times more potent than CoQ10 or idebenone, and has shown clinical efficacy in diverse mitochondrial respiratory chain deficiencies [67].

### *Malfunction of Mitochondrial Biogenesis via the SIRT1/PGC-1α/PPARγ Pathway: Therapeutic Implications*

In addition to the impairment of OXPHOS, significant mitochondrial depletion is found in the spinal cord of *Abcd1*⁻ mice and in the affected white matter of X-ALD patients [19, 38]. We unveil that *Abcd1*⁻ mice show a 50% reduction in mitochondrial DNA copy numbers concomitant with downregulation of the mitochondrial biogenesis pathway driven by PGC-1α/PPARγ, with diminished expression of the biogenesis factors NRF1 and TFAM, which negatively impact on the amounts of mitochondrial protein such as cytochrome c, NDUFB8 and VDAC. Moreover, an excess of VLCFA may play a role in this phenomenon, as subunits of complex III and IV of the ETC were decreased by C24:0 and C26:0 in the neuronal cell line SK-NB-E [53]. We believe that this reduction in mitochondrial amounts exerts an impact on the axonopathy exhibited in X-ALD for the reasons mentioned previously. Indeed, deletion of TFAM is characterized by decreases in both mitochondrial DNA and OXPHOS activity, which are correlated to axonal degeneration and gliosis [68].

To compensate for the defective mitochondrial biogenesis, we sought to stimulate the PGC-1α/PPARγ axis with an agonist of PPARγ, thus treating the X-ALD mice with the thiazolidinedione pioglitazone, which is widely used as antidiabetic drug [69]. In a preclinical test, pioglitazone satisfactorily restored redox and bioenergetic homeostasis, and halted axonal degeneration and associated locomotor disability [19]. The data lend support to repurposing pioglitazone for clinical trials with AMN patients and reveal novel molecular mechanisms of action of pioglitazone in neurodegeneration. Pioglitazone has recently been granted orphan drug designation for the treatment of adrenoleukodystrophy (EU/3/14/1245) and holds great potential for clinical translation.

Based on a parallel approach, we targeted the sirtuin 1 gene, a protein deacetylase that activates PGC-1α, and thus controls mitochondrial content among other functions related to bioenergetics, redox homeostasis and inflammation [70, 71]. We found that both transgenic overexpression of SIRT1 and drug treatment by the SIRT1 activator resveratrol normalize mitochondrial content in spinal cords of *Abcd1 null* mice, along with restoring respiration, redox and bioenergetic homeostasis, while preserving axonal health and locomotor capabilities [20].

However, the encouraging results obtained with pioglitazone and resveratrol do not allow us to discriminate between the benefits of a purely antioxidant therapy and a second strategy combining both improved biogenesis and amelioration of oxidative damage, which are most likely directly linked in this model.

### *Impact of C26:0 Excess on Proteasome Function*

The ubiquitin-proteasome system (UPS) is pivotal in the rapid clearance of damaged, misfolded or aggregated proteins in both healthy and diseased states, and has been shown to play a role in the degradation of oxidized proteins [72, 73]. Conformational diseases involving proteasome malfunction such as polyglutamine diseases, e.g. Huntington's disease and several spinocerebellar ataxias, tauopathies (e.g. AD and Pick's disease) and synucleinopathies (e.g. Lewy body disease), are associated with oxidative stress, and in most cases oxidative damage arises very early in the course of the pathology [57, 74]. Moreover, altered UPS activity has been observed in the brain from AD, PD and ALS patients [75]. Further, selective lack of 26S proteasome subunits in the substantia nigra results in a PD-like phenotype, whereas mice with depletion of 26S in spinal motor neurons exhibit an ALS-like phenotype [75], underscoring the central role of proteasomes in neurodegeneration. In X-ALD, we have detected chronic and progressive malfunctioning of the UPS resulting from the accumulation of oxidatively modified proteins, with some of them involved in bioenergetic metabolism. Furthermore, the immunoproteasome (i-proteasome) machinery appears, in the absence of overt inflammation, upregulated in response to redox imbalance. i-proteasomes are recruited to mitochondria when fibroblasts are exposed to an excess of C26:0, an adaptive action to oxidative stress. Finally, antioxidant treatment regulates proteasome expression while normalizing its function, preventing i-proteasome induction and its translocation to mitochondria. Our findings support a key role of i-proteasomes in the quality control of mitochondria during oxidative damage in X-ALD [35, 38]. Interestingly, rotenone, an inhibitor of mitochondrial complex I, and antimycin, an inhibitor of complex III, repress proteasome expression and activity. Finally, it has been demonstrated that UPS activity is reduced in fibroblasts from patients with mutations in complex I and complex IV of the respiratory chain [76]. Furthermore, increases in ubiquitin protein were correlated with decreases in UPS activity in *Ndufs4*$^{-/-}$ mice [77]. Altogether these data suggest that ETC dysfunction and/or mitochondrial ROS negatively regulate the UPS activity.

### *Defective Autophagic Flux: mTOR Inhibition as a Therapeutic Target*

How to stimulate proteasome activity? Along with degradation by proteasomes, autophagy constitutes the major route for eliminating misfolded or modified intracellular proteins [78]. We, therefore, reasoned that induction of autophagy in X-ALD could be a plausible strategy to compensate for proteasome impairment by increasing clearance of oxidized proteins. However, using the *Abcd1*$^{-}$ mouse model, we detected an impairment of autophagic flux in spinal cords. The mechanism appeared to be an aberrant activation of the mTOR (mammalian target of rapamycin) pathway by VLCFA excess. We, thus, used a specific activator of autophagy through inhibition of mTOR, the rapamycin ester *temsirolimus,* currently in clinical use as anticancer agent [79, 80], to successfully block mTOR signaling, restore autophagic flux and arrest axonal degeneration [17]. Interestingly, temsirolimus action preserved proteasome function, and redox and metabolic homeostasis with conserved ATP and NADH production [17]. Thus, activating autophagy is sufficient to correct oxidative damage, which indicates that autophagic flux may be considered as an internal antioxidant defense system. These findings provide first evidence linking impaired autophagy to X-ALD, thus providing a valuable therapeutic target and an FDA-approved compound (*temsirolimus*) ready to be evaluated and translated into the clinics.

There is a direct link between ROS produced at the mitochondrial OXPHOS site and autophagy [81]. Indeed, rotenone, the inhibitor of mitochondrial complex I, decreases autophagic flux, causing lysosomal vacuoles to accumulate in SH-SY5Y cells [82]. Antimycin A, the inhibitor of mitochondrial complex III, acts as a specific autophagy blocker, lowering LC3-II levels [83].

The autophagy process is altered in other neurodegenerative disorders such as AD and Huntington's disease. In these cases, autophagic flux is impaired, the number of autophagic vacuoles increases, and autophagic substrates accumulate in affected tissues [57, 84]. Impaired autophagolysosome formation, which is characterized by increased p62 as well as decreased LC3-II and mTOR activation, is evidenced in Duchenne's muscular dystrophy, just as we observed in X-ALD. This effect was due to chronic oxidative stress produced by NADPH oxidase in *mdx* mice [85]. Chronic oxidative stress is a hallmark of aging and may be a major contributing factor to the well-known decline of autophagy in aging, and thus may be a major culprit in cellular accumulation of waste and aggregated proteins in neurodegenerative disorders.

## Concluding Remarks

Compelling evidence indicates that X-ALD recapitulates the pathological hallmarks of the main neurodegenerative disorders, with intertwined peroxisomal, mitochondrial, proteasomal and autophagy dysfunction. Neutralization of ROS prevents these alterations along with axonal degeneration, which suggests that oxidative stress is a major culprit in this disease. Boosting biogenesis of new, intact mitochondria, together with enhancing clearance of damaged mitochondria by mitophagy or by the proteasome, holds therapeutic potential for this particular peroxisomal disease, but also for other multifactorial or inherited disorders in which axonal degeneration is at the bulk of clinical symptoms.

X-ALD, a rare monogenic peroxisomal disorder, may constitute a suitable paradigm to dissect molecular mechanisms and altered pathways in neurodegeneration, and thus a model to uncover new disease-modifying treatments that may also help in other, more prevalent neurodegenerative diseases.

## Acknowledgment

This study was supported by grants from the European Leukodystrophy Association [ELA2012-033C1], the Spanish Institute for Health Carlos III [FIS PI11/01043, FIS PI14/00410, FIS ICI14/00076], the Oliver's army, the Hesperia Foundation and the Autonomous Government of Catalonia [2009SGR85, 2014SGR1430] to A.P. The CIBER on Rare Diseases (CIBERER) and the CIBER on Neurodegenerative Diseases (CIBERNED) are initiatives of the ISCIII.

## References

1 Berger J, Forss-Petter S, Eichler FS: Pathophysiology of X-linked adrenoleukodystrophy. Biochimie 2014;98:135–142.

2 Engelen M, Kemp S, Poll-The BT: X-linked adrenoleukodystrophy: pathogenesis and treatment. Curr Neurol Neurosci Rep 2014;14:486.

3 Ferrer I, Aubourg P, Pujol A: General aspects and neuropathology of X-linked adrenoleukodystrophy. Brain Pathol 2010;20:817–830.

4 van Roermund CW, Visser WF, Ijlst L, van Cruchten A, Boek M, Kulik W, Waterham HR, Wanders RJ: The human peroxisomal ABC half transporter ALDP functions as a homodimer and accepts acyl-CoA esters. FASEB J 2008;22:4201–4208.

5 Wiesinger C, Kunze M, Regelsberger G, Forss-Petter S, Berger J: Impaired very long-chain acyl-CoA β-oxidation in human X-linked adrenoleukodystrophy fibroblasts is a direct consequence of ABCD1 transporter dysfunction. J Biol Chem 2013;288:19269–19279.

6 Fourcade S, Ruiz M, Camps C, Schluter A, Houten SM, Mooyer PA, Pampols T, Dacremont G, Wanders RJ, Giros M, et al: A key role for the peroxisomal ABCD2 transporter in fatty acid homeostasis. Am J Physiol Endocrinol Metab 2009;296:E211–E221.

7 Sandlers Y, Moser AB, Hubbard WC, Kratz LE, Jones RO, Raymond GV: Combined extraction of acyl carnitines and 26:0 lysophosphatidylcholine from dried blood spots: prospective newborn screening for X-linked adrenoleukodystrophy. Mol Genet Metab 2012;105:416–420.

8 Turgeon CT, Moser AB, Morkrid L, Magera MJ, Gavrilov DK, Oglesbee D, Raymond K, Rinaldo P, Matern D, Tortorelli S: Streamlined determination of lysophosphatidylcholines in dried blood spots for newborn screening of X-linked adrenoleukodystrophy. Mol Genet Metab 2015;114:46–50.

9 Engelen M, Kemp S, de Visser M, van Geel BM, Wanders RJ, Aubourg P, Poll-The BT: X-linked adrenoleukodystrophy (X-ALD): clinical presentation and guidelines for diagnosis, follow-up and management. Orphanet J Rare Dis 2012;7:51.

10 Aubourg P, Chaussain JL: Adrenoleukodystrophy: the most frequent genetic cause of Addison's disease. Horm Res 2003;59(suppl 1):104–105.

11 Engelen M, Barbier M, Dijkstra IM, Schur R, de Bie RM, Verhamme C, Dijkgraaf MG, Aubourg PA, Wanders RJ, van Geel BM, et al: X-linked adrenoleukodystrophy in women: a cross-sectional cohort study. Brain 2014;137:693–706.

12 Aubourg P, Blanche S, Jambaque I, Rocchiccioli F, Kalifa G, Naud-Saudreau C, Rolland MO, Debre M, Chaussain JL, Griscelli C, et al: Reversal of early neurologic and neuroradiologic manifestations of X-linked adrenoleukodystrophy by bone marrow transplantation. N Engl J Med 1990;322:1860–1866.
13 Cartier N, Aubourg P: Hematopoietic stem cell transplantation and hematopoietic stem cell gene therapy in X-linked adrenoleukodystrophy. Brain Pathol 2010;20:857–862.
14 Gong Y, Mu D, Prabhakar S, Moser A, Musolino P, Ren J, Breakefield XO, Maguire CA, Eichler FS: Adeno-associated virus serotype 9-mediated gene therapy for X-linked adrenoleukodystrophy (X-ALD). Mol Ther 2015;23:824–834.
15 van Geel BM, Poll-The BT, Verrips A, Boelens JJ, Kemp S, Engelen M: Hematopoietic cell transplantation does not prevent myelopathy in X-linked adrenoleukodystrophy: a retrospective study. J Inherit Metab Dis 2015;38:359–361.
16 Aubourg P, Adamsbaum C, Lavallard-Rousseau MC, Rocchiccioli F, Cartier N, Jambaque I, Jakobezak C, Lemaitre A, Boureau F, Wolf C, et al: A two-year trial of oleic and erucic acids ('Lorenzo's oil') as treatment for adrenomyeloneuropathy. N Engl J Med 1993;329:745–752.
17 Launay N, Aguado C, Fourcade S, Ruiz M, Grau L, Riera J, Guilera C, Giros M, Ferrer I, Knecht E, et al: Autophagy induction halts axonal degeneration in a mouse model of X-adrenoleukodystrophy. Acta Neuropathol 2015;129:399–415.
18 Lopez-Erauskin J, Fourcade S, Galino J, Ruiz M, Schluter A, Naudi A, Jove M, Portero-Otin M, Pamplona R, Ferrer I, et al: Antioxidants halt axonal degeneration in a mouse model of X-adrenoleukodystrophy. Ann Neurol 2011;70:84–92.
19 Morato L, Galino J, Ruiz M, Calingasan NY, Starkov AA, Dumont M, Naudi A, Martinez JJ, Aubourg P, Portero-Otin M, et al: Pioglitazone halts axonal degeneration in a mouse model of X-linked adrenoleukodystrophy. Brain 2013;136:2432–2443.
20 Morató L, Ruiz M, Boada J, Calingasan NY, Galino J, Guilera C, Jové M, Naudi A, Ferrer I, Pamplona R, et al: Activation of sirtuin 1 as therapy for the peroxisomal disease adrenoleukodystrophy. Cell Death Differ 2015, Epub ahead of print.
21 Forss-Petter S, Werner H, Berger J, Lassmann H, Molzer B, Schwab MH, Bernheimer H, Zimmermann F, Nave KA: Targeted inactivation of the X-linked adrenoleukodystrophy gene in mice. J Neurosci Res 1997;50:829–843.
22 Chaudhry V, Moser HW, Cornblath DR: Nerve conduction studies in adrenomyeloneuropathy. J Neurol Neurosurg Psychiatry 1996;61:181–185.
23 Dumser M, Bauer J, Lassmann H, Berger J, Forss-Petter S: Lack of adrenoleukodystrophy protein enhances oligodendrocyte disturbance and microglia activation in mice with combined Abcd1/Mag deficiency. Acta Neuropathol 2007;114:573–586.
24 Pujol A, Hindelang C, Callizot N, Bartsch U, Schachner M, Mandel JL: Late onset neurological phenotype of the X-ALD gene inactivation in mice: a mouse model for adrenomyeloneuropathy. Hum Mol Genet 2002;11:499–505.
25 Pujol A, Ferrer I, Camps C, Metzger E, Hindelang C, Callizot N, Ruiz M, Pampols T, Giros M, Mandel JL: Functional overlap between ABCD1 (ALD) and ABCD2 (ALDR) transporters: a therapeutic target for X-adrenoleukodystrophy. Hum Mol Genet 2004; 13:2997–3006.
26 Ferrer I, Kapfhammer JP, Hindelang C, Kemp S, Troffer-Charlier N, Broccoli V, Callyzot N, Mooyer P, Selhorst J, Vreken P, et al: Inactivation of the peroxisomal ABCD2 transporter in the mouse leads to late-onset ataxia involving mitochondria, Golgi and endoplasmic reticulum damage. Hum Mol Genet 2005;14:3565–3577.
27 Lu JF, Barron-Casella E, Deering R, Heinzer AK, Moser AB, deMesy Bentley KL, Wand GS, McGuinness MC, Pei Z, Watkins PA, et al: The role of peroxisomal ABC transporters in the mouse adrenal gland: the loss of Abcd2 (ALDR), not Abcd1 (ALD), causes oxidative damage. Lab Invest 2007;87:261–272.
28 Muneer Z, Wiesinger C, Voigtlander T, Werner HB, Berger J, Forss-Petter S: Abcd2 is a strong modifier of the metabolic impairments in peritoneal macrophages of ABCD1-deficient mice. PLoS One 2014; 9:e108655.
29 Weber FD, Weinhofer I, Einwich A, Forss-Petter S, Muneer Z, Maier H, Weber WH, Berger J: Evaluation of retinoids for induction of the redundant gene ABCD2 as an alternative treatment option in X-linked adrenoleukodystrophy. PLoS One 2014; 9:e103742.
30 Berger J, Pujol A, Aubourg P, Forss-Petter S: Current and future pharmacological treatment strategies in X-linked adrenoleukodystrophy. Brain Pathol 2010; 20:845–856.
31 Fourcade S, Ruiz M, Guilera C, Hahnen E, Brichta L, Naudi A, Portero-Otin M, Dacremont G, Cartier N, Wanders R, et al: Valproic acid induces antioxidant effects in X-linked adrenoleukodystrophy. Hum Mol Genet 2010;19:2005–2014.
32 Pujol A, Troffer-Charlier N, Metzger E, Chimini G, Mandel JL: Characterization of the adrenoleukodystrophy-related (ALDR, ABCD2) gene promoter: inducibility by retinoic acid and forskolin. Genomics 2000;70:131–139.

33 Singh J, Khan M, Singh I: Caffeic acid phenethyl ester induces adrenoleukodystrophy (Abcd2) gene in human X-ALD fibroblasts and inhibits the proinflammatory response in Abcd1/2 silenced mouse primary astrocytes. Biochim Biophys Acta 2013; 1831:747–758.

34 Fourcade S, Lopez-Erauskin J, Galino J, Duval C, Naudi A, Jove M, Kemp S, Villarroya F, Ferrer I, Pamplona, R, et al: Early oxidative damage underlying neurodegeneration in X-adrenoleukodystrophy. Hum Mol Genet 2008;17:1762–1773.

35 Launay N, Ruiz M, Fourcade S, Schluter A, Guilera C, Ferrer I, Knecht E, Pujol A: Oxidative stress regulates the ubiquitin-proteasome system and immunoproteasome functioning in a mouse model of X-adrenoleukodystrophy. Brain 2013;136:891–904.

36 Lopez-Erauskin J, Galino J, Bianchi P, Fourcade S, Andreu AL, Ferrer I, Munoz-Pinedo C, Pujol A: Oxidative stress modulates mitochondrial failure and cyclophilin D function in X-linked adrenoleukodystrophy. Brain 2012;135:3584–3598.

37 Lopez-Erauskin J, Galino J, Ruiz M, Cuezva JM, Fabregat I, Cacabelos D, Boada J, Martinez J, Ferrer I, Pamplona R, et al: Impaired mitochondrial oxidative phosphorylation in the peroxisomal disease X-linked adrenoleukodystrophy. Hum Mol Genet 2013;22:3296–3305.

38 Schluter A, Espinosa L, Fourcade S, Galino J, Lopez E, Ilieva E, Morato L, Asheuer M, Cook T, McLaren A, et al: Functional genomic analysis unravels a metabolic-inflammatory interplay in adrenoleukodystrophy. Hum Mol Genet 2012;21:1062–1077.

39 Mastroeni R, Bensadoun JC, Charvin D, Aebischer P, Pujol A, Raoul C: Insulin-like growth factor-1 and neurotrophin-3 gene therapy prevents motor decline in an X-linked adrenoleukodystrophy mouse model. Ann Neurol 2009;66:117–122.

40 Singh I, Pujol A: Pathomechanisms underlying X-adrenoleukodystrophy: a three-hit hypothesis. Brain Pathol 2010;20:838–844.

41 Wang Y, Yang J, Yi J: Redox sensing by proteins: oxidative modifications on cysteines and the consequent events. Antioxid Redox Signal 2012;16:649–657.

42 Pamplona R, Barja G: Highly resistant macromolecular components and low rate of generation of endogenous damage: two key traits of longevity. Ageing Res Rev 2007;6:189–210.

43 Fourcade S, Lopez-Erauskin J, Ruiz M, Ferrer I, Pujol A: Mitochondrial dysfunction and oxidative damage cooperatively fuel axonal degeneration in X-linked adrenoleukodystrophy. Biochimie 2014;98:143–149.

44 Galea E, Launay N, Portero-Otin M, Ruiz M, Pamplona R, Aubourg P, Ferrer I, Pujol A: Oxidative stress underlying axonal degeneration in adrenoleukodystrophy: a paradigm for multifactorial neurodegenerative diseases? Biochim Biophys Acta 2012; 1822:1475–1488.

45 Powers JM, Pei Z, Heinzer AK, Deering R, Moser AB, Moser HW, Watkins PA, Smith KD: Adrenoleukodystrophy: oxidative stress of mice and men. J Neuropathol Exp Neurol 2005;64:1067–1079.

46 Vargas CR, Wajner M, Sirtori LR, Goulart L, Chiochetta M, Coelho D, Latini A, Llesuy S, Bello-Klein A, Giugliani R, et al: Evidence that oxidative stress is increased in patients with X-linked adrenoleukodystrophy. Biochim Biophys Acta 2004;1688:26–32.

47 Galino J, Ruiz M, Fourcade S, Schluter A, Lopez-Erauskin J, Guilera C, Jove M, Naudi A, Garcia-Arumi E, Andreu AL, et al: Oxidative damage compromises energy metabolism in the axonal degeneration mouse model of X-adrenoleukodystrophy. Antioxid Redox Signal 2011;15:2095–2107.

48 Rhein V, Song X, Wiesner A, Ittner, LM, Baysang G, Meier F, Ozmen L, Bluethmann H, Drose S, Brandt U, et al: Amyloid-beta and tau synergistically impair the oxidative phosphorylation system in triple transgenic Alzheimer's disease mice. Proc Natl Acad Sci U S A 2009;106:20057–20062.

49 Gispert S, Ricciardi F, Kurz A, Azizov M, Hoepken HH, Becker D, Voos W, Leuner K, Muller WE, Kudin AP, et al: Parkinson phenotype in aged PINK1-deficient mice is accompanied by progressive mitochondrial dysfunction in absence of neurodegeneration. PLoS One 2009;4:e5777.

50 Baarine M, Andreoletti P, Athias A, Nury T, Zarrouk A, Ragot K, Vejux A, Riedinger JM, Kattan Z, Bessede G, et al: Evidence of oxidative stress in very long chain fatty acid – treated oligodendrocytes and potentialization of ROS production using RNA interference-directed knockdown of ABCD1 and ACOX1 peroxisomal proteins. Neuroscience 2012;213:1–18.

51 Baarine M, Ragot K, Athias A, Nury T, Kattan Z, Genin EC, Andreoletti P, Menetrier F, Riedinger JM, Bardou M, et al: Incidence of Abcd1 level on the induction of cell death and organelle dysfunctions triggered by very long chain fatty acids and TNF-alpha on oligodendrocytes and astrocytes. Neurotoxicology 2012;33:212–228.

52 Hein S, Schonfeld P, Kahlert S, Reiser G: Toxic effects of X-linked adrenoleukodystrophy-associated, very long chain fatty acids on glial cells and neurons from rat hippocampus in culture. Hum Mol Genet 2008;17:1750–1761.

53 Zarrouk A, Vejux A, Nury T, El Hajj HI, Haddad M, Cherkaoui-Malki M, Riedinger JM, Hammami M, Lizard G: Induction of mitochondrial changes associated with oxidative stress on very long chain fatty acids (C22:0, C24:0, or C26:0)-treated human neuronal cells (SK-NB-E). Oxid Med Cell Longev 2012; 2012:623257.

54 Li Y, Zhao Y, Yu W, Jiang S: Scavenging ability on ROS of alpha-lipoic acid (ALA). Food Chemistry 2004;84:563–567.

55 Sancheti H, Kanamori K, Patil I, Diaz Brinton R, Ross BD, Cadenas E: Reversal of metabolic deficits by lipoic acid in a triple transgenic mouse model of Alzheimer's disease: a 13C NMR study. J Cereb Blood Flow Metab 2014;34:288–296.
56 Lin MT, Beal MF: Mitochondrial dysfunction and oxidative stress in neurodegenerative diseases. Nature 2006;443:787–795.
57 Martinez A, Portero-Otin M, Pamplona R, Ferrer I: Protein targets of oxidative damage in human neurodegenerative diseases with abnormal protein aggregates. Brain Pathol 2010;20:281–297.
58 Fernandez-Checa JC, Fernandez A, Morales A, Mari M, Garcia-Ruiz C, Colell A: Oxidative stress and altered mitochondrial function in neurodegenerative diseases: lessons from mouse models. CNS Neurol Disord Drug Targets 2010;9:439–454.
59 Court FA, Coleman, MP: Mitochondria as a central sensor for axonal degenerative stimuli. Trends Neurosci 2012;35:364–372.
60 Kruska N, Schonfeld P, Pujol A, Reiser G: Astrocytes and mitochondria from adrenoleukodystrophy protein (ABCD1)-deficient mice reveal that the adrenoleukodystrophy-associated very long-chain fatty acids target several cellular energy-dependent functions. Biochim Biophys Acta 2015;1852:925–936.
61 Whitcomb RW, Linehan WM, Knazek RA: Effects of long-chain, saturated fatty acids on membrane microviscosity and adrenocorticotropin responsiveness of human adrenocortical cells in vitro. J Clin Invest 1988;81:185–188.
62 Ho JK, Moser H, Kishimoto Y, Hamilton JA: Interactions of a very long chain fatty acid with model membranes and serum albumin. Implications for the pathogenesis of adrenoleukodystrophy. J Clin Invest 1995;96:1455–1463.
63 Giorgio V, von Stockum S, Antoniel M, Fabbro A, Fogolari F, Forte M, Glick GD, Petronilli V, Zoratti M, Szabo I, et al: Dimers of mitochondrial ATP synthase form the permeability transition pore. Proc Natl Acad Sci U S A 2013;110:5887–5892.
64 Fransen M: Cyclophilin D: a therapeutic target to counteract reactive oxygen species-mediated damage in neurodegenerative disease? Brain 2012;135: 3525–3526.
65 Rao VK, Carlson EA, Yan SS: Mitochondrial permeability transition pore is a potential drug target for neurodegeneration. Biochim Biophys Acta 2014; 1842:1267–1272.
66 Morato L, Bertini E, Verrigni D, Ardissone A, Ruiz M, Ferrer I, Uziel G, Pujol A: Mitochondrial dysfunction in central nervous system white matter disorders. Glia 2014;62:1878–1894.
67 Enns GM, Kinsman SL, Perlman SL, Spicer KM, Abdenur JE, Cohen BH, Amagata A, Barnes A, Kheifets V, Shrader WD, et al: Initial experience in the treatment of inherited mitochondrial disease with EPI-743. Mol Genet Metab 2012;105:91–102.
68 Sorensen L, Ekstrand M, Silva JP, Lindqvist E, Xu B, Rustin P, Olson L, Larsson NG: Late-onset corticohippocampal neurodepletion attributable to catastrophic failure of oxidative phosphorylation in MILON mice. J Neurosci 2001;21:8082–8090.
69 Pfutzner A, Weber MM, Forst T: Pioglitazone: update on an oral antidiabetic drug with antiatherosclerotic effects. Expert Opin Pharmacother 2007;8: 1985–1998.
70 Donmez G: The neurobiology of sirtuins and their role in neurodegeneration. Trends Pharmacol Sci 2012;33:494–501.
71 Paraiso AF, Mendes KL, Santos SH: Brain activation of SIRT1: role in neuropathology. Mol Neurobiol 2013;48:681–689.
72 Dennissen FJ, Kholod N, van Leeuwen FW: The ubiquitin proteasome system in neurodegenerative diseases: culprit, accomplice or victim? Prog Neurobiol 2012;96:190–207.
73 Goldberg AL: Protein degradation and protection against misfolded or damaged proteins. Nature 2003; 426:895–899.
74 Nunomura A, Hofer T, Moreira PI, Castellani RJ, Smith MA, Perry G: RNA oxidation in Alzheimer disease and related neurodegenerative disorders. Acta Neuropathol 2009;118:151–166.
75 McKinnon C, Tabrizi SJ: The ubiquitin-proteasome system in neurodegeneration. Antioxid Redox Signal 2014;21:2302–2321.
76 Segref A, Kevei E, Pokrzywa W, Schmeisser K, Mansfeld J, Livnat-Levanon N, Ensenauer R, Glickman MH, Ristow M, Hoppe T: Pathogenesis of human mitochondrial diseases is modulated by reduced activity of the ubiquitin/proteasome system. Cell Metab 2014;19:642–652.
77 Song L, Cortopassi G: Mitochondrial complex I defects increase ubiquitin in substantia nigra. Brain Res 2015;1594:82–91.
78 Martinez-Vicente M, Cuervo AM: Autophagy and neurodegeneration: when the cleaning crew goes on strike. Lancet Neurol 2007;6:352–361.
79 Bove J, Martinez-Vicente M, Vila M: Fighting neurodegeneration with rapamycin: mechanistic insights. Nat Rev Neurosci 2011;12:437–452.
80 Dancey JE: Therapeutic targets: mTOR and related pathways. Cancer Biol Ther 2006;5:1065–1073.
81 Morales CR, Pedrozo Z, Lavandero S, Hill JA: Oxidative stress and autophagy in cardiovascular homeostasis. Antioxid Redox Signal 2014;20:507–518.

82 Mader BJ, Pivtoraiko VN, Flippo HM, Klocke BJ, Roth KA, Mangieri LR, Shacka JJ: Rotenone inhibits autophagic flux prior to inducing cell death. ACS Chem Neurosci 2012;3:1063–1072.

83 Ma X, Jin M, Cai Y, Xia H, Long K, Liu J, Yu Q, Yuan J: Mitochondrial electron transport chain complex III is required for antimycin A to inhibit autophagy. Chem Biol 2011;18:1474–1481.

84 Wong E, Cuervo AM: Autophagy gone awry in neurodegenerative diseases. Nat Neurosci 2010;13:805–811.

85 Pal R, Palmieri M, Loehr JA, Li S, Abo-Zahrah R, Monroe TO, Thakur PB, Sardiello M, Rodney GG: Src-dependent impairment of autophagy by oxidative stress in a mouse model of Duchenne muscular dystrophy. Nat Commun 2014;5:4425.

Aurora Pujol, MD, PhD, ICREA Professor
Laboratory of Neurometabolic Diseases
Institut d'Investigació Biomèdica de Bellvitge (IDIBELL)
L'Hospitalet de Llobregat
ES–08908 Barcelona (Spain)
E-Mail apujol@idibell.cat

# Author Index

# Subject Index